MANAGEMENT OF EMOTIONAL PROBLEMS IN MEDICAL PRACTICE

CONTRIBUTORS

KARL M. BOWMAN, M.D.
Medical Superintendent, The Langley Porter Clinic; Professor of Psychiatry, University of California Medical School, San Francisco; Past President, American Psychiatric Association.

FRANCIS J. GERTY, M.D.
Professor and Head, Department of Psychiatry, Director, Psychiatric Division, Neuropsychiatric Institute, University of Illinois College of Medicine; Senior Attending Psychiatrist St. Luke's Hospital; Chairman Deans' Subcommittee on Psychiatry, Veterans Administration Hospital, Hines, Illinois.

LEWIS L. ROBBINS, M.D.
Director, Department of Adult Psychiatry, The Menninger Foundation, Topeka, Kansas.

FRANKLIN G. EBAUGH, M.D.
Clinical Professor of Psychiatry, University of Colorado; formerly Director of Colorado Psychopathic Hospital and Professor of Psychiatry and Head of the Department at the University of Colorado.

OTTO BILLIG, M.D.
Associate Professor of Psychiatry, Vanderbilt University School of Medicine; Psychiatrist-in-Chief, Out-patient Department Vanderbilt University Hospital, Nashville.

GEORGE C. HAM, M.D.
Professor and Chairman, Department of Psychiatry, University of North Carolina, School of Medicine; Chief of Service, North Carolina Memorial Hospital, Chapel Hill, North Carolina.

LEO H. BARTEMEIER, M.D.
Medical Director, Seton Psychiatric Institute, Baltimore; Teaching Analyst, Washington Psychoanalytic Institute, Clinical Professor of Psychiatry, Georgetown University Medical School, Washington, D.C. Past President, American Psychiatric Association.

WALTER C. ALVAREZ, M.D.
Professorial Lecturer in Medicine, Emeritus, University of Illinois College of Medicine; Consultant in Medicine, Emeritus, Mayo Clinic; Editor-in-Chief, Modern Medicine, Geriatrics; Editorial Board of other journals and newspapers.

MARC H. HOLLENDER, M.D.
Associate Professor, Department of Psychiatry, University of Illinois College of Medicine; Staff Member, Institute for Psychoanalysis, Chicago.

Management of

EMOTIONAL PROBLEMS

in Medical Practice

Edited by

SAMUEL LIEBMAN, M.D.

Medical Director, North Shore Health
Resort, Winnetka, Ill.; Clinical Assistant
Professor of Psychiatry, University of Illi-
nois College of Medicine

Philadelphia   Montreal

J. B. LIPPINCOTT COMPANY

Distributed in Great Britain by

PITMAN MEDICAL PUBLISHING CO., LIMITED

London

Library of Congress
Catalog Card Number 56-10802

PRINTED IN THE UNITED STATES OF AMERICA

PREFACE

The physician's responsibility to his patient extends beyond the treatment of ailing organs. With each appointment the medical practitioner is confronted by a different personality with its problems of emotional as well as physical adjustment. The doctor cannot realistically compartmentalize his thinking and therapeutic efforts to treat only part of the person. To render the best service he must have the background and insight to view the human organism as a whole.

It is not feasible to encompass all of our knowledge, limited as it is, within the confines of one thin volume. However, assistance can be offered to the medical man who deals with all types of emotional problems in his everyday practice. It is hoped that the publication of these lectures will serve this end.

This volume is the second in a series based on lectures given at the North Shore Health Resort. The chapters consist of the material presented by the authors during our Sixth Annual Lecture Series titled "Psychiatric Problems in Medical Practice." Each talk was geared to present a practical approach to the management of emotional problems seen in the everyday care of patients by the medical practitioner.

Assisting patients in the solution of emotional problems not only promotes better health for them but is of direct value to their families and to the community. One of our aims is to make some contribution to such efforts. To further this aim the Board of Directors of the North Shore Health Resort and each of the authors have assigned all royalties that accrue from the sale of this monograph to the American Psychiatric Association for use in the promotion of better emotional health.

It is hoped that the professional readers of this volume will be stimulated to raise questions and make suggestions as to the type of material that would be useful to them in their function as physicians. We welcome communications on such matters as a guide for the development of further lecture series.

SAMUEL LIEBMAN, M.D.

CONTENTS

1

PSYCHIATRIC EMERGENCIES

Karl M. Bowman, M.D.

In line with some of the popular books, this paper might have as its subtitle, "What To Do Before the Psychiatrist Comes." It is not easy to say just what we mean by psychiatric emergencies. Since psychiatry infiltrates all the other branches of medicine, all emergencies may be called psychiatric, at least in part. It is worth emphasizing that there are important psychiatric implications in many emergencies and difficult situations which are not generally recognized. In these, the psychiatrist has more to contribute than is generally thought to be the case. Practically, we may say psychiatric emergencies are where the psychiatrist has something of importance to contribute, where he might be called to assist in the care of the patient, or where at least the understanding of the psychiatrist's method of dealing with such problems would enable the general practitioner to deal with the situation in a more efficient and helpful fashion. It is difficult to make a classification of these emergencies, so I have taken them up pretty much in the manner in which they have occurred to me.

Since psychiatry is the special field of medicine concerned with the mental functioning and the behavior of the individual, psychiatric emergencies might be defined as those emergencies which occur particularly to the mental functioning and behavior of the individual. The psychiatrist can be of service to the general medical man when patients show these disorders in mental functioning and behavior. Some of the most common situations are suicidal tendencies, depressions, threats, assaults, antisocial behavior, drug poisoning, delirium and excitements. A great many physicians become rather panicky when confronted with such problems, and seek to get out of the situation as quickly and easily as possible. If a patient is labeled as a psychiatric case, many feel that this

1

diagnosis precludes the general medical man having charge of the case or even having anything to do with it. I hope that my discussion this evening may help to alleviate some of the anxiety which many physicians feel when confronted with some of these problems, and that the general practitioner will realize that there are many conditions labeled psychiatric which can be treated by the general practitioner. The label of psychiatric does not automatically mean that the patient should be locked up and kept away from the rest of medical cases.

It is well to emphasize that the majority of patients with mental disorders are seen first by a doctor who is not a psychiatrist and it is, therefore, important for the rest of the medical profession to have some general understanding of psychiatric diagnosis, what precautions are necessary and what treatment is indicated. The first and often the most difficult decision is, can the general practitioner treat this patient by himself, should he call in a psychiatrist as a consultant, or should he turn him over completely to a psychiatrist?

SUICIDAL IMPULSE

Suicide is an important cause of death, and for every successful suicide there are probably at least five or ten unsuccessful attempts. This is a problem which comes up before the general practitioner quite frequently. A patient threatens to do away with himself. Immediately we hear the statement that any patient who threatens to kill himself will not do it but is merely trying to get attention and sympathy. There is just enough truth in this statement that it can lead to serious harm, since everyone with much experience in psychiatry has had numerous patients who have threatened suicide and have then carried it out. Many neurotic patients who are toying with the idea do not really intend to commit suicide, but occasionally they are suddenly overwhelmed with such extreme emotion that they do make a very genuine and, at times, successful attempt at suicide, or, again, an individual may be placed in a certain position where suicide is the only way of saving face and he gives way to the impulse. There are also a few genuine accidents where a patient who does not seriously intend to commit suicide, but is making a dramatic appeal for attention and sympathy, actually ends up by killing himself. Some cases may represent the real subconscious impulse for suicide conquering, and therefore the reason for the death of the patient, but I believe there are some cases where it is really a genuine accident. Every case of depression should be looked upon as a potential suicide and the doctor should consider whether it is fair to the patient and to the family to allow the patient to remain at home or in a relatively unprotected environment. In any case, the whole situation should be gone over in detail with the family and they should be asked to accept joint responsibility for whatever plan of treatment is agreed upon. It is manifestly impossible and it is not desirable to put every patient with any suicidal tendencies in an institution. We speak of a calculated risk which is taken in such cases, and even with the best of psychiatric advice the so-called calculated risk occasionally becomes a miscalculated risk. If there is any question of doubt in the mind of the general practitioner, he should avail himself of psychiatric consultation. Many times a frank discussion with the patient himself, pointing out these risks, the need of protecting him against himself and asking his help in the whole matter, will cause the patient to discuss his feelings quite frankly and fully and will indicate to what degree one can take risks.

When patients make threats of suicide it is very difficult to make a calm, judicial appraisal of the situation. The family is likely to go to one extreme or the other. They may refuse to see that the patient is seriously sick—they maintain the suicide threat is not a serious one, they act as if the doctor were trying to harm the patient by getting him into a hospital in a more protected situation, and they interpose every possible objection to hospitalizing the patient, who is quite sick mentally and a serious suicidal risk. It is well to remember that these are the families who will be most disturbed and accusatory if things do go wrong and the patient does make a successful suicidal attempt. So while I would agree that it is most unpleasant to try to convince such families of the necessity of hospitalization, I would point out that the situation will be infinitely more unpleasant if the doctor does not do so and a disaster occurs. It should be emphasized that the well-designed psychiatric hospital is a much safer place for the suicidal patient than his own home, where there is commonly the possibility of jumping out a window, turning on the gas, taking various poisons which are present in the kitchen or the bathroom, stabbing himself with some sharp, pointed kitchen instrument, electrocuting himself, or drowning himself in the bathtub. Psychiatric hospitals are designed to prevent the occurrence of any of these situations. Families commonly say, "But doctor, how can he get well in this hospital with all these crazy people about him?" The answer to this is that the patient got sick in his own home and that a large percentage of patients do get well in psychiatric hospitals. Many times patients are more at ease when they are away from their family. This is apparently true of many senile patients, who, in their own homes, feel they must direct and control everything, but who settle down quietly and accept the directions of the doctors and nurses. So frequently does this occur that it has led to the idea on the part of many persons that a lot of old persons are being railroaded into the hospital by relatives who want to get rid of them or get their money.

Threats of suicide are one of the most common emergencies which the general practitioner faces. No such threats should be disregarded and considerable time must be spent in evaluating the seriousness of such threats. It is important to remember that even those who do not seriously intend to commit suicide often miscalculate, take an overdose of some drug or, when turning the gas on, anticipate the arrival of someone else, also make a mistake. According to George N. Thompson, 50 per cent of patients with involutional melancholia attempt suicide and about 25 per cent are successful.

The agitated depression who is overactive is the more serious suicidal risk than the slowed-up, retarded depression, who finds everything, including a suicidal attempt, too much for him to undertake. When one has a patient with an agitated depression walking around, wringing his hands, expressing many somatic or nihilistic delusions, extremely self-accusatory, it is obvious that here we have a most serious suicidal risk and that a psychiatric hospital is the best place for such a patient. Early morning is often the most dangerous time from the standpoint of suicide. The depression is most severe at that time as the patient faces the prospect of another impossible day ahead. Characteristically, in many depressions, the degree of depression becomes less as the day wears on, and some patients who start out extremely depressed in the morning may be fairly cheerful by nightfall, only to show the recurrence of their depression the following morning.

Arteriosclerotic depressions must be considered as very serious suicidal risks. Most patients with cerebral arteriosclerosis appreciate that their intellectual capacities are decreasing and that physically they are on the downgrade. It is obvious to them, and correctly so, that arteriosclerosis is a progressive condition, that no cure exists and hence, the treatment of such depressions is much more difficult than either the manic-depressive depressions or the involutional melancholias, where one knows that the condition is primarily self limited and that in the manic-depressive even without electroshock treatment over 90 per cent will make a complete recovery.

Many of the depressions with cerebral arteriosclerosis respond well to electroshock treatment. The newer drugs, chlorpromazine and reserpine, are valuable in some cases, particularly where there is high blood pressure. The problem facing the patient is, however, the inevitable one of all aging persons, that man does not live forever, and that with increased age comes the decrease in both physical and mental powers. Some persons are able to accept this and do not have serious conflicts over the whole matter. Others, however, are unable to face the inevitable situations of life and are inclined to take matters into their own hands, even when not particularly depressed. They may prefer to not wait for the inevitable breakdown.

The patient with schizophrenia is often unpredictable, which is one of the reasons that so many suicides do occur in schizophrenic patients. Such a possibility is most difficult to anticipate, and a brief casual interview with the patient often fails to disclose the danger.

Many persons suffering with prolonged and often incurable conditions, such as cancer, decide that it is better to do away with themselves than to continue suffering. This decision may be in a setting of depression or it may be a fairly judicial appraisal on the part of the individual that life is no longer worth living. The newspapers record a steady succession of such cases occurring among persons of great prominence. All physicians should be aware of the frequency of suicidal attempts among such cases, even though there may be no warning symptoms. It is difficult to do much in the way of prevention in such cases; however, the use of drugs or even lobotomy may lessen the dangers in certain cases, and the whole management of the patient's life with careful supervision may also help prevent the occurrence of such tragedies.

Alcoholics often go through a quite severe depression following drinking bouts and times when they are faced with the fact that their attempts to discontinue alcohol have met with serious failure. These are commonly rather transient depressions, but quite serious ones. In all cases where suicide seems a danger, the matter must be discussed thoroughly with responsible members of the family and a decision as to the course of action to be taken should be reached, with responsibility being carried jointly by the family and the physician. In case of doubt it is always better to err on the side of safety and have the patient placed in a well-run psychiatric institution where there will be the best possible precautions taken against self-injury. Even then it is well to realize that it is not possible to produce an institution that will be 100 per cent safe for suicidal patients, and that the intelligent, alert patient bent on suicide is extremely likely to carry out his attempt no matter what the situation is in which he is placed. One has merely to point to the three successful attempts at suicide made at the time of the Nuremberg trials where the German prisoners were placed in single cells under 24-hour-a-day observation by a special guard, who, when not present in the cell with the prisoner, was peering through a peephole in the door.

Obviously, the best precaution against suicide is to place the patient in a well-run institution with a special nurse assigned for 24-hour observation. In general, in such an institution, it is better to have the suicidal patients in a ward and under the constant observation of a nurse, rather than to place them in single rooms where they will be more isolated and have more opportunities to carry out their self-destructive tendencies.

A second situation, somewhat similar to this, is where the patient has made an unsuccessful attempt at suicide and has been brought into the hospital. When I was at Bellevue we had an average of 15 patients a day brought to the psychiatric ward following some sort of suicidal attempt. The question that comes up immediately is, will this patient repeat this attempt if he is allowed to go out, or is the situation now so changed that there is no serious risk in allowing him to leave the hospital? Some cases are self-evident. A young married woman turns on the gas when she hears her husband unlocking the front door. He comes in and finds her lying stretched out on the kitchen floor, with the odor of gas. The patient is taken to the hospital—it is found that she has inhaled very little gas and that physically there is no need for any special treatment. A brief questioning shows that there has been one of the usual marital quarrels, the husband is remorseful and full of good promises, the wife has gotten her own way and there is no immediate danger of another suicidal attempt. Such a patient can be allowed to go home quite safely, but if any patient resorts to gestures to this degree following quarrels with her husband there should be some sort of psychiatric study and treatment, because sometime in the future the situation may get worse and a more serious attempt may occur.

It is well recognized that many unsuccessful suicide attempts relieve the tension; that the patient feels that God or fate has intervened to prevent his death, and he is at least temporarily satisfied to go on as he is. One is faced, therefore, with the necessity of estimating the tensional relief that a patient has derived from a suicidal attempt or gesture. It is obvious that such patients may have recurrences of their suicidal tendencies, but it is neither practical nor desirable to segregate such persons for the rest of their natural lifetimes because they may sometime make another suicidal attempt which may be successful.

THE VIOLENT PATIENT

Another situation, where the question of injuring others and not himself is the problem, imposes even greater difficulties. The doctor may be called in because some patient is threatening harm to some other member of the family or to some outsider. At times, the patient may be armed. The whole situation is an extremely difficult and dangerous one. Sometimes the patient is very noisy, shouting and making a great scene, but at other times he is sitting there very quietly and is in good contact with his surroundings. The family physician may be the one person that the patient can trust. It may be possible for him to sit down and talk the matter over with the patient alone. Occasionally, the psychiatrist will be able to get the patient to talk over the whole situation. This is, perhaps, one of the first and best approaches to make. If someone can get the patient talking about the whole situation, if someone can sit and listen to him quietly, it may be that the patient will talk things out and in many cases it is possible to work out a satisfactory solution. The doctor will have to figure what risks he wishes to take and when he should turn matters over to the police. At a certain stage this is the only way of dealing with the situation.

Acts of violence may be carried out by patients with various types of disorder. The epileptic furor is one such condition. In coming out of an epileptic convulsion, certain patients go into a state of furor in which they may violently attack any person near them, and in a few cases an actual sexual assault may also be attempted. These are commonly quite transient attacks and the patient must be temporarily forcibly restrained. Usually the condition passes off inside of a few minutes. Occasionally it is quite prolonged and the use of intravenous barbiturates may be very valuable in helping control the condition.

While many patients who are under the influence of alcohol become very surly and belligerent, there are cases which are commonly spoken of as pathologic intoxication and in which the patient goes through a wild excitement, much like the epileptic furor. Either suicidal or homicidal impulses may express this, and the patient is most difficult to handle. Here the use of 5 cc. of a 10 per cent solution of metrazol intravenously may work in almost miraculous fashion. In one such case that was brought to Bellevue when I was there, a man made a sudden unprovoked assault on the people near him at the Pennsylvania Station. It took six policemen to subdue him and bring him to Bellevue, where he was still fighting and struggling. Metrazol was injected intravenously, taking about 35 seconds so as not to produce a convulsion. I saw the patient about 15 minutes later. He was completely clear, and showed no abnormal impulses. He talked quietly and coherently, he had no memory of what had happened and expressed surprise when told what had occurred. This was about 5 o'clock in the afternoon. The patient ate a good supper, went to bed and slept quietly during the night without hypnotics, and was discharged the next morning.

The patient with delirium tremens is commonly a suicidal risk rather than a homicidal risk. He often tries to get away from the visual hallucinations of a terrific character and will go headfirst out of the window or attack persons he sees as individuals who are preventing him from escaping from the terrifying animals that he sees approaching him.

The patient with acute alcoholic hallucinosis, on the other hand, is very dangerous. Unlike the delirium tremens patient, who is confused and shows signs of an organic delirium, the acute alcoholic hallucinosis patient usually has a very clear sensorium, but commonly hears voices of a threatening character. In order to protect himself, he may attack others and at times will get a gun and shoot at the persons he believes are trying to harm him. A number of innocent persons have been killed by attacks of this sort. It is obvious, therefore, that with the diagnosis of delirium tremens, acute alcoholic hallucinosis or pathologic intoxication with homicidal or suicidal tendencies, the patient should be placed under medical care and put in a psychiatric institution. The ordinary alcoholic who is extremely belligerent likewise should be controlled.

REFUSAL TO EAT

The general practitioner at times faces the problem of patients who refuse to eat, often with great loss of weight and the danger of death from starvation. This may occur in babies and small children and go through all age groups, including the seniles. The problem with small children is commonly an emotional situation when the child easily discovers that he can upset and control his parents by refusal to eat. After organic disease is ruled out, the method of handling the patient is fairly clear to the psychiatrist. Many cases respond to so-called "therapeutic neglect." If the parents are no longer concerned and leave the child to his own devices, the child often will eat in a quite satisfactory manner. Other cases are, of course, much more complicated and require careful psychiatric treatment, often taking considerable time. One of the most difficult of cases to deal with is that of anorexia nervosa. Much has been written about this condition, and it is not always easy to differentiate from actual disease of the pituitary. The typical case is an adolescent girl, often with a better-looking or more favored sister as a rival. At times there are definite difficulties between father and mother which are sensed by the child and there may even be rivalry with the mother. In a few cases the adolescent girl has been overweight and tries to reduce by eating less, until she finally gets into a very emaciated condition. Early recognition of such a case is important and there is no simple formula for treatment. Threats of forcible feeding or actual forcible feeding should never be resorted to, except as a final measure where life itself is threatened. Many cases respond very well to prolonged intensive psychotherapy which commonly includes treatment of other members of the family as well.

Refusal to eat occurs in certain types of well-known psychoses. The patient with a severe depression may have lost all interest in life and may even voluntarily refuse to eat as an attempt to commit suicide. In catatonic stupors in schizophrenia, patients likewise may refuse to swallow and to take any liquid or food. Certain organic cases may also do the same. In these cases immediate forced feeding is desirable, and it is important that the feeding have an excess of vitamins and minerals, as well as a high protein content. Since only a limited amount can be given at a single tube feeding, it is often desirable to insert a Levine tube and to give small amounts every half-hour or hour, so that one ends with having given the individual a large amount of fluid. It is well to remember that a salt deficiency often occurs and that the giving of salt stimulates the sense of thirst on the part of the patient as well as the ability to retain fluid. In patients with acute delirium one may sometimes pour a little orange juice on the lips and in the mouth so that the patient gets the taste. For most persons, orange juice is pleasant tasting and a number of delirious patients will swallow orange juice if one gives it very slowly, either from a cup or tube, or even by taking a teaspoon and spilling a spoonful at a time in the mouth.

DRUG INTOXICATION

A delirium due to drugs is another situation in which the help of the psychiatrist may be asked. It is well to remember two things —one, that in general a normal person does not develop a drug delirium because he seldom receives drugs in sufficient dosage to produce such a delirium; and two, that drug deliria are often due to a mixture of drugs so that the physician looking for a clear-cut picture of a single drug may be confused and not realize the true nature of the condition. For example, an alcoholic, who is perhaps a somewhat abnormal individual to begin with, uses large amounts of alcohol, takes barbiturates to help him sleep at night and amphetamine to wake him up in the morning, and finally develops a delirious picture which does not seem to conform clearly to any single drug intoxication. All organic pictures are modified by the personality of the patient, and this individual reaction to various drugs must always be borne in mind. Some persons are excited by taking morphine, instead of the usual effect. Bromide intoxication is probably less common than it used to be, but is often missed by the physician because he looks for a bromide rash and there is none present. It is important to remember that most cases of bromide delirium do not show the typical bromide rash, and the diagnosis can only be confirmed by a history of large doses of bromides or a blood bromide examination. The treatment of bromide delirium is, of course, the treatment of all deliria, with the giving of large amounts of salt so that the chlorides will replace bromides.

Acute and chronic barbiturate intoxications are conditions that the general practitioner has to deal with. Acute barbiturate intoxication is most commonly the result of a suicidal attempt. It, therefore, has psychiatric elements in it. In the acute condition, respiratory failure is the greatest danger. Various drugs, such as metrazol, are recommended, and the use of the electric stimulator, as developed in some of the electric shock machines, is of great value. The stomach should be washed out immediately and general symptomatic treatment employed. As the patient recovers the psychiatric aspect of the whole problem will become evident and the case should then be managed in the same fashion as any other unsuccessful attempt at suicide.

Chronic barbiturate poisonings at first may give the appearance of a serious organic brain disease, but the presence of the neurologic signs of nystagmus, marked tremor, ataxia, with thick speech and occasional ankle clonus and Babinski, together with the mental picture of an organic coma, should at once cause the physician to suspect barbiturate poisoning. The diagnosis should be confirmed by the history and determination of blood barbiturates. An abrupt and complete withdrawal of barbiturates may throw the patient into convulsions; therefore, the physician should try to find out what dosage the patient has been taking and give just enough barbiturates to prevent the occurrence of convulsions, but as soon as possible stop any further giving of barbiturates. This will probably be a matter of a week or ten days. Delirium may occur during the withdrawal period, with hallucinations and a good deal of confusion. The patient may be restless and unable to sleep. After the patient has recovered from the effects of the drug, a careful study as to the cause of his use of drugs should be made and then appropriate treatment instituted, which would be the usual psychiatric attempt to figure out the patient's personal problems and what can be done to help him solve them, so that he will no longer need to rely upon drugs.

Ordinarily, when the physician is called in to see a patient who is disturbed, restless and perhaps noisy, he is inclined to give some sedative drug. If the patient does not respond well the physician is likely to increase the dosage of this drug, and in a number of cases an actual drug delirium is produced. At this stage the psychiatrist is often called in and he may be able to diagnose this and point out that complete withdrawal of all drugs is the proper treatment, not giving still more drugs.

For patients who are overactive, excited and delirious, morphine is not a good drug. It may be pointed out further that morphine raises intracranial pressure and often masks signs of an associated intracerebral or intra-abdominal injury. There is an old saying that morphine not only puts the patient to sleep but also the physician. Paraldehyde is probably the safest drug we have for such conditions. Alcoholics seem to enjoy its most unpleasant taste and any doubt as to the diagnosis disappears if the patient takes the dose of paraldehyde and gulps it down with obvious satisfaction.

Two new drugs have recently received great attention for the treatment of acute emotional disorders. These are chlorpromazine and reserpine, both of value, but the reports at the present time are so contradictory that it does not appear worthwhile to spend much time trying to clarify this whole situation. One point seems evident, that two cases with the same appearance respond very differently—one patient responds beautifully to either of these drugs, quiets down and shows marked improvement; another patient shows no improvement or perhaps seems worse after the use of either or both of these drugs. This unpredictability of beneficial results has not been explained, and in our present stage of knowledge one probably has simply to try out the drug and see what effect he gets. The dangers should be carefully estimated, particularly the fall in blood pressure with reserpine and the possible jaundice with chlorpromazine.

COMPLICATIONS OF PREGNANCY

A number of conditions in relation to pregnancy may call for the services of a psychiatrist. Vomiting of pregnancy often has a large psychological element in it, and in any case of a pregnant woman where vomiting seems to have gone beyond ordinary amounts, psychological factors should be thoroughly investigated. In a number of cases it is surprising how a few interviews in which the patient is encouraged to talk out all her feelings and fears about pregnancy will result in the disappearance of these symptoms.

The extreme vomiting of pregnancy may reach a point where the life of the mother is threatened and where the question of therapeutic abortion comes up. In all such cases a psychiatric study is indicated and may result in alleviation of the symptoms. One extreme condition that has come up a number of times is where a woman threatens suicide if a therapeutic abortion is not done. Here we have a situation in which psychiatric help obviously is needed. The answer may depend in part on the patient's religious beliefs, as well as what is legal. For example, is a woman who has been forcibly raped and impregnated, who seriously states that she will kill herself if an abortion is not done, entitled to such an operation? To what extent is the life and permanent health of the mother threatened if one does not carry out such an operation? Such cases are very complicated, and no general rule can be laid down. Each case must have a careful psychiatric examination before any decision is made.

HYSTERIA

One not uncommon condition which is difficult to treat is the so-called acting out or acute hysteria. The patient, usually a woman, is quite excited, often full of complaints and accusations, noisy, unco-operative, and the family demand that something be done at once. Since these episodes frequently occur in the middle of the night they are the bane of all physicians, and it is not easy to get immediate psychiatric consultation. Two approaches are suggested: One, that the physician accept the idea that he is going to spend one, two or three hours with the patient; that he sit down, encourage her to talk, listen attentively and indicate sympathetic understanding by his attitude. Many times such a patient will talk herself out after a while, quiet down and go to sleep. The other treatment is an injection of one of the sleeping drugs in sufficient dosage to knock the patient out. It is well to remember, however, that some of these excited and disturbed patients do not react as does the ordinary patient, and will require massive doses to overcome the emotional state. Psychiatric treatment is indicated as soon as the patient is able to receive psychotherapy.

PANIC

Individual or mass states of panic constitute a psychiatric emergency. When the Japanese bombed Chungking, the Chinese had excellent caves in which to take refuge when bombings occurred. However, there were times when panic reactions in these caves caused hundreds of deaths, whereas the bombings caused almost none.

Two recent articles deal with emergency situations studied by competent psychiatrists. In 1951, a severe flood occurred in Topeka, Kansas. Dr. W. C. Menninger reported "Psychological Reactions in an Emergency (Flood)" in the August 1952 issue of the *American Journal of Psychiatry*. He notes the reactions of volunteer workers not personally affected and the reactions of victims and describes the changing attitudes from the beginning, through the crisis and the great letdown after everything was over except continuing care of victims and cleaning up. In the November 1952 issue of the *American Journal of Psychiatry*, Dr. Richard D. Loewenberg of Bakersfield, California, wrote on "Psychological Reactions in an Earthquake." Space does not permit giving details of the reactions to these two catastrophes, but any discussion of psychiatric emergencies must include a discussion of catastrophes of these types.

Treatment may be summed up as follows: The emergency treatment of panic conditions will depend in part on the reaction of the patient. Where the panic reaction is individual, and there is no danger of infecting others, there is much less immediate need of drastic treatment and immediate alteration of the patient's condition. Where, however, one is confronted with the question of mass panic, immediate steps must be taken to prevent the spread of this reaction. We know that panic reactions are among the most contagious conditions there are and prevention is the most important thing. As far as possible one should talk to the patient and isolate him from others, if there is any possible way of doing this. Under such conditions the treatment of the patient is the same as in any other acute emotional state. The doctor must himself set an example of self-control. He must be interested in the patient's condition. Ordinarily, a punitive type of treatment is not good. In a few cases, a patient who is starting to scream or become violent may be stopped by slapping his face vigorously, swearing at him, or some treatment of that sort. This, however, is not generally desirable and can, in many cases, do great harm. The patient should be encouraged to talk things out, he should be reassured and he may be offered a cigarette, a drink of coffee, or any food and drink available, as a way of getting him to do something and taking his mind off his problems. In some cases it is desirable to give the patient a strong sedative. In other cases he should be gotten back into activities as soon as possible and joined up with the group. Experience with war neurosis shows that patients should be seen as near the battle line as possible and as quickly as possible. Some immediate treatment should be given, and the attitude of the doctor will be of the greatest importance in determining whether or not the patient is able to conquer his feelings. As soon as possible the patient should be returned to the front. Any prolonged period of invalidism away from the front greatly decreases the chances of returning the patient to active duty.

From the standpoint of treating a group of individuals in an incipient panic state (or where a few are already beginning to show it), as might well occur in threats of bombing, a number of points can be kept in mind. If an organized and preferably uniformed group can move in and take charge at once, the populace commonly will accept such control and direction and this will greatly aid in preventing panic. The people should be put to work of some sort. People with nothing to do except anticipate danger or death tend to become more upset and panicky. The individual who is occupied in some constructive way works out some of his emotions and is much less likely to break. It is important that the individual feels that he is one of a group, that he belongs; therefore, the quick organization of the populace into groups, with persons to take charge, will accomplish much in panic prevention. The fear of the unknown is commonly greater than the fear of the known. If the individuals can get some clear understanding of the situation they will usually behave better. The prevention of panic, before such threats as bombing, is by organization, education, drilling, etc., of the groups. When people know just what they are supposed to do and what is expected of them, the minute an alarm sounds they are likely to go ahead and carry out the duties which have been given to them. Motivation and leadership are two of the important factors in preventing mass panic. The problem of the therapist is to enable an emotionally disturbed person to again face difficult and disturbing situations and to function in a reasonably effective manner. Brief periods of rest, isolation, with food and drink provided, are of the greatest value. All treatment should be given with the implied idea that the patient is incapacitated for only a very brief period of time and that he will shortly recover and function at his usual level. A doctor must be most careful against implanting any idea that the patient is not going to recover.

2

THE USE AND ABUSE OF SEDATIVES
AND STIMULANTS

Francis J. Gerty, M.D.

THE HUMAN BEHAVIOR BACKGROUND

Human beings seek comfort. In the very beginning of their lives they seem to take comfort for granted and complain by one means or another, usually by voice or other action, when they are uncomfortable. In infancy the comfort, at first accepted but later sought, is of a sensual kind—warmth, relaxation, freedom of movement, no obstruction to healthy functioning, comfortably full stomach, sleep and, probably from the beginning, some need for very real physical closeness to others. Throughout life each of these matters will have its importance to every one of us. There will be individual variations in the degree of that importance and many varieties of transformation and substitution of the desired satisfactions will occur. We shall continue to wish for comfort, positively when we seek joyful exhilaration, negatively when we try to avoid or fly from pain, tension, anxiety or fear.

Beginning early in life the preponderantly physical demands for comfort have others added to them, ones connected less to the bodily part of our personalities. In our personal connections, there is desire for comfortable, full and satisfying acceptance by others. The fulfillment of this desire is soon opposed by the rules and misrules of social life, the prohibitions, reasonable and unreasonable, which our seniors believe necessary to impose. By and large these rules are probably good enough, but not always, and even when good their application can be more painful than a new pair of stiff shoes to a bare foot which has been accustomed to freedom of movement. These seniors, often hitherto the fountains of our comfort, take on a new behavior which gives us pause, hurts and

17

leads us to protest. We seem to invite the display of this new and unexpected attitude more and more frequently, and in an increasing variety of situations.

There is also within us early in life an irrepressible urge to explore exuberantly and with satisfying release of energy. This energy is our motive power. We need it to go places and do things and will need it all through life. It is a positive endowment, an élan vital, the possession of which will always be desired. Yet, it can bring us into distressing predicaments—physical discomfort for one thing and other discomforts not easily localized in any bodily organ or area. These discomforts can make us unhappy all over. As discomforts are fearful to endure, we strive vigorously to escape them. One must escape from himself to succeed in escaping from some of them.

In infancy when we didn't succeed in finding desired comforts and joys or were hurt by the hard rules of life, we found certain remedies and set certain habit patterns which will remain with us in some measure throughout life. Probably the first remedy for most of us was the warm, comforting enfoldment in a mother's arms. Failing this, perhaps, there was the sobbing refuge in sleep, maybe using our first placebos, a favored blanket or a strongly sucked thumb. Again sometimes there was physical flight, running away from home to an outer world where all feelings would be reduced to a more satisfactory common denominator than the difficult odd fractions one had to deal with in the home. Sometimes, after many failures to find better means, there was a flight into a phantasy world where things were made to be as one liked them. Of course, the most satisfactory way to deal with discomfort and tension is the means we can all still wish to attain for our own use—learning to avoid the extremes of pain by paying the fair price in personal inconvenience and patient endurance which represents a good and satisfactory bargain with life and the world. Wise and kindly guidance will be required if we are to learn the use of this means. Most of us have experimented with all of the other means before we have gained any success with using this one.

As long as life and consciousness endure, some elements of these five means of moving from the pole of discomfort toward that of comfort can be clearly discerned in every situation involving the distresses of illness or the difficulties and discomforts of ordinary living. As might be expected, the first two means, being the most fundamental and the most direct, will find their counterpart in the use of sedatives. With sedatives we seek immediate and positive results comparable to the refuge of mother's arms or that of sleep. Immediateness and positiveness of action take precedence over other considerations as is always the case in the face of emergency or supposed emergency. In this, too, we are often as impatient as children. In discussing the use and abuse of sedatives and stimulants, immediateness and positiveness of effect cannot alone be the objectives in prescribing. The positive seeking of high points of pleasure must be restrained by moderation. The relief from discomfort can never be as direct and uncomplicated as we might wish.

GENERAL PHARMACOLOGIC CONSIDERATIONS

It is now necessary to descend from the philosophic to the pharmacologic plane. The central nervous system depressants are far more important therapeutically than are the stimulants. They are probably the most widely used of all therapeutic agents. There are several important categories of central nervous system depressants—general anesthetics, sedatives, hypnotics, soporifics, narcotics, analgesics and antipyretics. The ones of chief interest to us in this discussion are sedatives, hypnotics or soporifics and narcotics. There is much overlapping in the meanings of these classificatory terms. For example, a sedative in large dose may become an anesthetic. Hypnotics produce a drug type of sleep which resembles but differs from normal sleep. Sedatives produce milder hypnosis, while calmed the patient is awake. Narcotics produce analgesia followed by pseudo sleep or stupor. Pain relief through the action of morphine exemplifies narcotic action. Analgesia is the relief of pain without stupefaction. The particular drugs which are of greatest importance in the depressant group are opium and its alkaloids, bromides, chloral hydrate, the barbiturates and paraldehyde. Extremely important because widely used, though not ordinarily prescribed, are alcohol and marijuana. Lately, several drugs known as tranquillizers, of differing chemical constitution but of somewhat similar actions, have been introduced. They include chlorpromazine, reserpine, Miltown and Frenquel. New ones are being added to the list rapidly. They have been in use only about three years and will receive only passing mention in this discussion. They are of a special class to which adequate attention is being given in the current literature.

In connection with the depressants, the matter of habituation, tolerance and dependence should be clarified as far as possible. Habituation is psychic and emotional dependence on a drug. Tolerance is the ability of the organism to accommodate itself to increased dosages of a drug. This increased tolerance is not developed to all drugs and we do not know why it is produced to any drug. The tolerance may be very far in excess of the dose required to prevent symptoms due to abstinence from a drug to which habituation has been established. By dependence is meant some measure of physiologic need for the continuance of a drug to which addiction has been established. Withdrawal of the drug causes abstinence symptoms, both psychic and physical. It is very difficult to determine the relative importance of these two sets of symptoms, the psychic and the physical. Studies of the pathologic and physical functional changes produced by the drugs in question or by their withdrawal has not helped our understanding of the whole problem very much. The psychic aspects and ramifications, being connected with the whole matter of human behavior, will certainly be complex. Hence, the preliminary philosophic remarks on some of the characteristics of human behavior at the beginning of this presentation. As always, the practitioner of medicine has the here and now treatment of the patient as his problem. He would be wisest to consider that problem as a whole. He should not dismiss withdrawal symptoms as being chiefly hysterical any more than he should regard them as being physical only.

The stimulants pose a different problem. In medical treatment the stimulants play a minor role in comparison with the depressants. They are intended to give a positive uplift of some kind, physical, mental or both. The central nervous system does not accept stimulation over a long period without being thrown into a state of depression. The stimulants also have numerous side effects and are not as selective in acting upon the nervous system as are the depressants. There are several that have important action on the central portion of the nervous system which should be mentioned. These are ephedrine, carbon dioxide, metrazol, picrotoxin, nicotine, caffeine, amphetamine and cocaine. Problems concerned with the use of some of these drugs will be discussed.

THE SEDATIVES

Until about a century ago the chief sedative hypnotic drugs employed in medicine were opium, alcohol and cannabis indica. In the next 50 years after that bromides, chloral hydrate, paraldehyde and barbiturate drugs were introduced into therapy in about the order given. All of these are definitely sedative and, in larger doses, hypnotic in their effects. All of them have been or are used widely in medical practice including psychiatric practice. When used with adequate knowledge of their action and with due caution, they can be of decided value. The very fact that they are valuable can lead by imperceptible steps to their abuse as remedies. Until 1857 none of them had been used extensively for sedative or hypnotic effects. All of the drugs mentioned acted most potently on the higher levels of the nervous system, particularly on the cerebral cortex. The most recent addition to our armamentarium, the tranquillizers, probably act on lower levels of the central nervous system since patients placed under their influence are easily aroused and mentally clear even after sleep has been produced by them. The limits of this paper will not permit much discussion of tranquillizing drugs such as chlorpromazine, reserpine, Miltown, Frenquel and others similar in action.

Opium. The name opium refers to the juice of the Oriental poppy, opium being the Greek word for juice. In the general uses of medicine, opium has been a drug of extreme importance for centuries. It has been and still is the sovereign analgesic. Its use as a remedy in psychiatric practice was less important than its use as a remedy in general medical practice. It has been of very great importance to psychiatrists, however, because it is a habit-forming drug and the treatment of addiction has been a problem for psychiatrists to manage not infrequently. Because of its effect in producing narcotic addiction, it has also been very important in connection with social problems generally and with national and international regulations concerning its manufacture, transportation and sale. Because its employment may lead to addiction, opium is a drug to be avoided rather than to be used in psychiatric practice. However, it has had a certain field of usefulness in the treatment of depressions. Before the days of convulsive therapy it was widely used for its calming effect and to allay psychic pain particularly in patients with agitated depressions. Here it was used in the form of powdered opium, pill of opium, or tincture of opium. The doses used to produce satisfactory effects were ordinarily large by present-day standards. Usually the equivalent of 4 to 8 gr. of powdered opium had to be used in the 24-hour period in divided doses in order to effect any result. It might be necessary to continue this treatment for months. Nevertheless, there seemed to have been no cases of addiction reported as a result of its use in this way probably because the dose was gradually reduced as the patient improved. In connection with the discussion of opium, a few remarks on the treatment of habituation to drugs will be in order.

Not infrequently, the psychiatrist is the physician consulted about the treatment of narcotic habituation. The literature dealing with narcotic addiction and its attempted regulation by governmental action is very large indeed. In the treatment of addiction the problem which receives the most attention, the immediate or emergency management of withdrawal symptoms is not actually the most important psychiatrically. While addiction can be produced by the treatment with narcotics of bona fide chronic painful illness, this is not the chief reason for the large addiction problem which we have to face. To the psychiatrist it is a question of what kind of a person becomes an addict rather than what the secondary effects of the addiction are on the person. Of course, the secondary consideration becomes of great importance in the actual management. The worse the primary problem is, the worse the secondary one will be. This is not the place to describe and discuss fully the ramifications of the addiction problem, nor, for that matter, its management in individual cases or through social and governmental means. If one observes the ordinary cautions and rules in prescribing opium and its derivatives and the synthetic analogues of these derivatives, there will be little danger of abuse of the prescription privilege in the course of ordinary psychiatric practice.

Alcohol by itself or in beverage form is rarely prescribed in psychiatric practice. I hardly need remark that a great deal of it is used. Psychiatrists generally regard its excessive use as a misguided and unconscious attempt at self-treatment by the user. As to primary causes and secondary effects, we must view alcohol addiction along the same general lines that apply in narcotic addiction. Management of the secondary effects cannot be the be-all and do-all of treatment. There was a time in the history of medicine, and this time is not much over a century ago, when alcohol had its important place in general practice and particularly in surgery. Prior to the discovery of chloroform and ether, heavy dosage with alcohol and opium was a not uncommon procedure as preparation for surgical operations. Self-treatment with alcohol is of still more ancient history.

Cannabis Indica. Along with alcohol and opium, cannabis indica, or indian hemp, must be regarded as one of the outmoded sedative hypnotic drugs. It has been known under various names, particularly the names of hashish and bhang. In action it was always undependable, being as much a deliriant as a sedative. Therapeutically it has dropped into disuse. Its chief importance at the present time is because of its extra-medical use by addicts in the form of marijuana. Of course marijuana is not prescribed. It is smoked illicitly by addicts in the form of cigarettes known also as "reefers." Treatment here again, in its psychiatric form at least, must be directed to the person rather than to the symptoms of the addiction. The immediate problem of treating the secondary effects is managed simply by the withdrawal of marijuana.

Bromides. Balard extracted bromine from sea water in 1826. Potassium bromide was introduced into the British Pharmacopoeia in 1835. However, it was not used at this time as a sedative, but was recommended as a substitute for iodides in the treatment of scrofula. It was soon noted that in this use there was also a sedative effect. At first the sedative effect was attributed to the potassium ion rather than to the bromide ion. In 1850 Huette made the first report on bromide intoxication. It was not until 1857 that Sir Charles Locock introduced bromides for sedative action. Actually, he was seeking an anaphrodisiac effect rather than a strictly sedative one. His reasoning was this: Many cases of epilepsy were thought to be due to onanism. It had been reported that potassium bromide had an anaphrodisiac effect. Therefore, bromides should be used to treat epilepsy. Locock reported 14 cases treated by bromides with good results except in one of them. The history of bromides in the treatment of epilepsy is very well known. Because of their other unpleasant effects in producing skin eruptions, mental dulling and bromide intoxication, their use has been practically superseded in epilepsy by newer remedies such as phenobarbital and dilantin. They are still used as sedatives by a good many physicians, and they are contained in many nostrums which can be purchased without a physician's prescription. Bromide salts can replace sodium chloride in the tissues. Bromides are excreted slowly and tend to accumulate in the body. If one is not cautious in the use of bromides, the cumulative effect may produce symptoms of delirium. There is a danger in treating patients who are already hyperactive, noisy and disturbed because of head injury or other medical or surgical conditions with bromides because the intoxication symptoms may become far more important than the ones which arose in connection with the original physical problem. It is my impression that the use of bromides in medicine is gradually diminishing. This is particularly true in psychiatric practice. A good rule to observe when one is called into consultation to see a delirious patient being treated for some physical condition is to have the blood bromide level determined. A blood bromide level of 125 to 175 mg. per cent often causes a bromide delirium. The treatment is simple but must be extended over a period of several weeks. It includes administration of sodium chloride and an adequate fluid intake. Of course the bromide medication must be withdrawn.

Chloral is a chlorinated derivative of ethyl alcohol. It is used in a hydrated form known as chloral hydrate. Chloral was first made by Liebig in 1832. It was not introduced into medicine until Liebrich used it in 1869. Liebrich wrongly thought that chloral was changed to chloroform in the body. This is the oldest of the truly hypnotic group of drugs. It is still one of the best but it had somewhat fallen into disuse. In recent years it has been used much more than it was 15 or 20 years ago. The sleep produced by it has a "natural" or "physiologic" appearance. The patient awakes with no great evidence of after-effect. There is a relatively low margin of safety between the adequate hypnotic dose and the minimum lethal dose. Ordinarily, between 15 and 30 gr. are used in a single dose. Death has occurred with doses as low as 40 gr. though the ordinary toxic dose is said to be between 100 and 150 gr. When chloral is mixed with alcohol, chloral alcoholate is formed. Chloral hydrate added to an alcoholic beverage constitutes the lengendary "knockout drops" or "Mickey Finn." Chloral hydrate has a decided value as a hypnotic though probably much less value as a sedative as its action is short.

Paraldehyde is a polymer of acetaldehyde. It was introduced into medicine in 1882 by Cervello. This is one of the most efficient and safe hypnotics that we have. Yet it has not been used as widely in private psychiatric practice as it has in the public psychiatric hospitals. It can be administered orally, intramuscularly or intravenously. For intramuscular and intravenous use it requires no sterilization preparation other than the aseptic measures that are used for the syringe and the skin. It does have a very pungent, disagreeable taste and odor. Many patients mistakenly call it formaldehyde though its odor is actually not as disagreeable as that of the antiseptic. It produces sleep very rapidly and the sleep is a profound one. In ordinary usage side-effects and after-effects are not very noticeable except that there is the clinging disagreeable odor which can be detected for from 12 to 24 hours after a dose has been administered. The taste is hard to disguise and sensitive stomachs do not tolerate the burning irritation of the medicine very well. Ordinarily, 4 to 6 cc. may be given intramuscularly and 4 cc. intravenously if injected slowly. It produces hypnotic effects very rapidly after injection. By mouth doses of 1 to 4 drams are not uncommon. Patients have survived doses of several ounces of paraldehyde. In spite of its disagreeable characteristics it is possible for people to become addicted to the use of this drug. Paraldehyde addicts are ones who wish to get an even quicker effect than alcohol will give them. Most of them are derived from the group of chronic alcoholics. When paraldehyde addiction occurs, its use as a remedy for the addict is contraindicated.

Barbiturates. By a wide margin the barbiturates are the drugs most used at the present time for sedation and hypnosis. The first of them, di-ethyl barbituric acid, or veronal, was introduced into medicine in 1903 by Fischer and von Mering. This was followed in 1910 by phenobarbital or Luminal. More than a score of barbiturates have been synthesized and introduced into medical use. Veronal was found to be cumulative in its action; phenobarbital less so. Most of the variants of the barbituric base have been synthesized with the idea of producing shorter acting drugs. One of the shortest acting is sodium pentothal which has been used in anesthesia and also for the type of psychiatric exploration under drug influence which came to be known as "narcosynthesis" during World War II. The barbiturates were also used in combination with other drugs in prolonged sleep therapy, "Dauerschlaf." Phenobarbital has had its most extensive use as an anticonvulsant in the treatment of epilepsy. Barbiturates have been combined with other drugs whose actions they may potentiate. Thus, it is not uncommon to combine them with analgesics. Another combination is with cerebral stimulants of the amphetamine group. The problem in using this combination is to find the patient whose needs are met with reasonable exactitude by two antagonistic drugs combined in the same pill in fixed dosage. Whether increased tension, sedation or a canceling out effect results is often somewhat open to question when such a combination is used. While the barbiturates potentiate the action of analgesics, the reverse is not true. However, with the tranquillizing drugs, chlorpromazine particularly, it is found that the barbiturate action is intensified very considerably. Therefore, one should be cautious in giving any barbiturates to a patient who is receiving chlorpromazine because the chlorpromazine may potentiate the action of the barbiturate so that much more marked effects are obtained from the barbiturates than had been anticipated. It is to be noted that the tranquillizing drugs may potentiate the action of alcohol also. It would be very difficult to estimate the extent to which barbiturates are used in medicine and used independently of prescription. While they should not be issued to patients except on prescription, my own observations lead me to believe that people obtain barbiturates far too easily and without prescription. The large number of barbiturates and their extensive sale indicate a very large per capita use. Unfortunately, the assurance to a patient that the medicine being prescribed is "harmless" may often lead that patient to take this expression altogether too literally. Certainly, there are far too many persons who think that a pill at bedtime is almost an absolute requirement and if one pill does not work, taking a second or even a third may be justified. Though theoretical arguments may be worked up easily about whether barbiturates are responsible for addiction or whether their use is characterized by tolerance and dependence factors such as appear with the opium derivatives, for practical purposes we must regard them as being drugs to which patients can become habituated. It is true that after habituation very large doses may not produce sleep even in a person who has no physical condition involving pain which would make him wakeful. Patients using such large doses and complaining of sleeplessness are often tense, irritable, and obviously emotionally disturbed. They may seem not to be confused and to function relatively normally intellectually. Nevertheless, after withdrawal, they are often unable to remember clearly what went on during the time they were taking large doses of barbiturates. During withdrawal, they may have convulsions and develop a confusional psychosis. In the treatment of withdrawal symptoms, usually a method of fairly rapid reduction is used. There seems to me to be unjustified fear of convulsions occurring during withdrawal. I do not mean to imply that convulsions will not occur. They are very likely to occur. In my own experience it has seemed that those patients who have had convulsions have made the best recoveries and have shown the least evidence of psychotic disturbance. This is in line with our experience in treating psychoses by the convulsion method. Consequently, I do not believe that we should hesitate to reduce the dose of barbiturate quite rapidly. In dealing with the whole problem of barbiturate habituation, we must focus our attention upon the person who is habituated rather than upon the secondary effects of the habituation. Contrariwise, when treating a patient with a psychiatric problem, we should be very wary of using barbiturates as adjuvants to psychotherapy.

cf P 11-12

THE STIMULANTS

Through the use of stimulants, an attempt is made to bolster or support the patient and urge him on to better and more satisfactory performance and feeling. With them we are seeking to promote values that are positive and active, whereas with sedatives we attempt to negate or diminish activities, tensions, and states of feeling that are unpleasant. In theory, stimulation might seem to be preferable to sedation. In practical use, the sedatives are far more important. The reasons have been pointed out already. To provide gentle, even, and continuous support to a patient through the use of stimulants is well nigh impossible. The fatigued, depressed patient with low energy endowment is commonly a frustrated and restless person. He is somewhat like the tired horse. He may be goaded into further action but the sources of his energy become still more depleted by the goading. The patient may be exhilarated for a time but as the exhilaration disappears, he experiences a feeling of increased tension and restlessness and he may find it difficult to sleep. As I have pointed out, the stimulants have many side-effects and their action on the central nervous system is not always primary. Prolonged stimulation of the central nervous system tends to exhaust and depress. There is a great variation in the action of the stimulants comparing one with another and also depending upon the dose and the mode of administration. The range of activity is from overcoming sleepiness through gentle exhilaration and increased activity up to convulsion. Stimulants are commonly used as emergency remedies to combat coma and states of shock. We call upon them particularly to combat the comas produced by sedatives. Others are used for special purposes such as the treatment of narcolepsy or the induction of convulsions for the treatment of psychoses.

Caffeine. The use of caffeine in general medical practice as a stimulant is very general. Its use in psychiatry, except in emergencies where physical support is required, is minimal. While it provides probably the simplest and evenest stimulation of the central nervous system of all of the stimulants, it is the enemy of sleep and sleeplessness is one of the common problems encountered in psychiatric practice.

Cocaine blocks nerve conduction; therefore, it serves as a local anesthetic in medical practice and was used formerly much more than it is now since many synthetic substitutes have been elaborated. It is also a very powerful stimulant to the central nervous system, but it is not used therapeutically for this purpose. Its dangers far outweigh its advantages. It is of interest to the psychiatrist chiefly because of the problem of cocaine addiction. Its use results in a peculiar kind of satisfaction, a euphoric excitement, sometimes accompanied by hallucinations which are pleasant in their content. The addict has a feeling of increased physical and mental strength. This addiction, therefore, is different from morphine addiction. The addict feels the gain of a positive stimulation and takes the drug for this effect, not as with morphine to avoid the symptoms of withdrawal. These effects of cocaine are very well known to addicts and it is obvious that this being the case, only persons with severe personality disorders are likely to become cocaine addicts. Also, as might be expected, the secondary effects make the personality disorders still more pronounced and complicate the problem of treatment.

Ephedrine and the Amphetamines (Benzedrine and Dexedrine). Ephedrine is an alkaloidal, active principle of plants belonging to the genus, Ephedra, particularly the Chinese herb known as Ma Huang. The active principle was isolated in 1885. It has an action somewhat similar to epinephrine. It was not used in western medicine until the late 1920's. Since then it has been used to relieve respiratory depression, cardiovascular allergic symptoms, and as an analeptic to treat narcolepsy and poisoning due to central depressant drugs. It was first used for the treatment of narcolepsy by Doyle and Daniels in 1930.

The amphetamines (Benzedrine and its longer-acting modification, Dexedrine) are widely used in psychiatric practice. The public and the general practitioner know of Benzedrine mostly through the use of the Benzedrine inhaler and the Benzedrine spray for nasal congestion. Both Benzedrine and Dexedrine are very potent stimulants to the central nervous system. The action of Benzedrine is sharper in its beginning and less prolonged than that of Dexedrine. Because of this, Dexedrine is replacing Benzedrine as a mood elevator. Nevertheless, it is to be noted that many people seem to have developed a Benzedrine inhaler habit, probably more for the stimulating effect than for the reduction of nasal congestion. These drugs also increase the blood pressure, a fact which must be borne in mind when administering them to patients with hypertension. Both drugs increase the metabolic rate; consequently, they have been used in weight-reducing programs. Unquestionably, these drugs are our best mood elevators at the present time. There are marked disadvantages to their use. The action begins quite rapidly but soon diminishes for a rapid downward curve in an hour or two. They are commonly given only during the morning hours because, if given later in the day, they may result in sleeplessness the following night. After the exhilaration passes, the patient often feels restless, edgy and tense. To cancel out this feeling of tension, the manufacturers combine Dexedrine with a barbituric acid derivative under the name of Dexamyl, but the difficulties of using such a preparation already have been alluded to under the discussion of the sedatives. In order to provide a more even distribution of the action over a longer period, the manufacturers also have put the drug out in the form of enteric-coated granules which dissolve at different times after administration, thus releasing a more uniform flow of the drug in graduated dosage. While the amphetamines produce a feeling of exhilaration and an impression in the subject that the mental efficiency is greater, there is no evidence that efficiency is actually increased. Some patients, particularly physicians, do become habituated to the use of the amphetamines, usually combining this habituation with a concomitant habituation to barbiturates, using the stimulant to keep awake in the daytime so that they can do their work and using the depressant in large enough doses to produce sleep at night. After using this combination for a while, the night and day cycle becomes completely disorganized and the general physical condition of the patient may suffer greatly. They should not be used indiscriminately in psychiatric disorders, but they do have some value in mild states of depression, but far less value in psychoneurotic conditions.

Metrazol and Picrotoxin. Metrazol stimulates the central nervous system strongly. It is a synthetic compound chemically related to camphor. Picrotoxin is obtained from *Cocculus indicus* or fish berries. It, too, is a powerful stimulant to the central nervous system. Both, being analeptic, are used in the treatment of barbiturate coma. Metrazol is historically important in psychiatry because of its use by Meduna in 1934 to treat psychoses through the production of convulsion in the psychotic patient. Since the introduction of the electroconvulsive method, it is not much used for this purpose nowadays. Picrotoxin has also been used for this purpose but the convulsive reaction is a delayed one and the drug never had much vogue for the purpose. Metrazol has been used by oral administration in attempts to increase the mental efficiency of elderly and arteriosclerotic persons. Opinions differ as to its value for this purpose.

The Tranquillizers. But little comment is required here on the tranquillizers, chlorpromazine, reserpine, Frenquel, Equanil and others. The current literature is replete with reports on the clinical experience with these drugs. They have been heralded with great acclaim as "wonder drugs" which promise to empty the wards of our public mental hospitals. It is too soon to really judge their merits. While relatively little is known as to their site of action in the nervous system, it seems quite certain that the cortex is but little affected because patients who have dropped off to sleep after the use of the tranquillizing drugs are usually mentally alert immediately upon being awakened. Patients who show evidence of defective liver function should not be given chlorpromazine. In some patients, reserpine produces depression, almost indistinguishable from essential depressions. They are very useful in states of excitement, particularly manic excitement. The calming effect even in small doses on elderly, anxious patients is especially noteworthy. Patients, initially anxious, are often made more so by their resulting feeling of tension. Since the tranquillizers reduce this feeling of tension, that part of the anxiety which originates secondarily is also relieved. It is very questionable that the tranquillizing drugs do anything to the inner causes of anxiety. Since the tension is reduced, it is thought that the patient is somewhat more amenable to psychotherapy.

GENERAL REMARKS AND CONCLUSIONS

When the physician is considering the prescription of a sedative, stimulant, or tranquillizing drug for any patient and particularly for a psychiatric patient, he faces a complex rather than a simple problem. All of the factors involved must be weighed in reaching his decision. The patient asks chiefly for quick and lasting relief from the symptoms that distress him, but the physician cannot accomplish his task so simply and directly. His knowledge of drugs and their pharmacology will not be sufficient. The problems of diagnosis and repeated re-evaluation of the patient, his disease or disorder, and the circumstances under which treatment is conducted must be ever in mind if the treatment is to be on a firm foundation. The drug is a physical remedy. The patient is more than a physical body to be acted upon by that remedy. He is a man with a history and a future. If it can possibly be avoided, the hospital patient should not be sent home still requiring a night sedative for sleep. The office patient should not be transformed into a hospital one by the too free and uncontrolled use of the prescription.

THE MANAGEMENT OF THE
ANXIOUS PATIENT

Lewis L. Robbins, M.D.

Man, because of his capacity not only to remember the past but to anticipate the future, is uniquely prone to suffer from anxiety. It is very possible that the entire history of civilization could be written from the standpoint of man's many efforts to eliminate or minimize anxiety. This is expressed in the superstitions of the ancients as well as in the prayers of modern man; in the works of the philosophers as well as in man's efforts to control the forces of nature and eliminate the dangers of disease. Man is ever probing into the unknown, not only to better understand the universe around him but also to anticipate and thus eliminate dangers that confront him.

It is not abnormal to worry about things which threaten our safety or our ideals or our plans. It is because of this capacity to see ahead and anticipate certain dangers and to avoid them that man has achieved what he has. There is, however, a significant difference between worry, fear and anxiety. Fear is related to something of which the individual is definitely and consciously aware. It is normal to be frightened when one is almost run over by a speeding automobile or is confronted with the business end of a gunman's revolver. Anxiety, however, is the result of a psychological conflict. Even though there may be some apparent external or reality events that precipitate it, the real cause of anxiety is not conscious. It is an expression of a conflict between instinctual needs and an environment that is unable or unwilling to gratify the needs. It may also be said to be the result of a failure of the integrative functions of the ego of the individual to discharge effectively instinctual energy or to erect adequate defenses against

33

instinctual drives. The stresses, whether they be from within or without, are temporarily at least beyond the ego's capacity to manage them and control them.

Much of the focus of attention of modern psychiatry has been devoted to the exploration of the meaning of anxiety and how the organism defends itself against it. Anxiety has been viewed as a signal or warning that something is wrong psychically, just as pain serves as a warning that something is wrong physically. Despite the disabling effects that may accompany anxiety the organism is usually still able to act in its own behalf even though outside help may be needed. If anxiety should become overwhelming then the condition of panic occurs. At such times the individual appears to be no longer able to defend himself. There is a transitory ego rupture which may become persistent.

SYMPTOMS OF ANXIETY

Anxiety is an unpleasant affect, an emotion or feeling tone. The individual may complain of feelings of apprehension, uneasiness, dread, fear or panic. Or he may be more aware of the physiologic concomitants such as tachycardia, dyspnea, sweating or some other somatic dysfunctions. An elevated systolic blood pressure, pupillary dilatation, fatigue and sleeping and eating disturbances may also be observed. Anxiety is experienced both mentally and physically and the patient may be suffering severely. Patients often attribute their anxiety to something organic or to some external danger. However realistic this may seem to be to the patient and to others, what he is really afraid of is never that which he thinks he is afraid of. The true cause is not conscious. Many who know nothing about psychopathology know that chronic worriers have never the slightest idea of the real thing they are worrying about. The phobias of children and many adults are obviously unrealistic, a fact which often the patient himself may recognize even though he is unable to control his feeling.

Every physician in the course of his regular professional activities encounters anxious patients. All patients, regardless of the nature of their presenting complaints, have some anxiety. It is well known that many physical complaints are either substitutes for or concomitants of anxiety. Because physicians often encounter patients who become anxious when they develop an organic illness, the fact that there are usually underlying emotional conflicts which the illness may have aroused is easily overlooked. To worry about one's illness is normal; in fact at times it might be abnormal not to do so. But anxiety as the term is used here is never normal and needs appropriate consideration. Any kind of illness may stimulate anxiety. An illness may create considerable disturbance not only to the individual but also to his family. In its mildest form it temporarily upsets plans. If more serious, major readjustments may be required. The duration and course of an illness may be unpredictable so that the patient and those around him are confronted both by threat and uncertainty. The nature of the illness, its course, the possible outcome, that is, whether the patient will recover at all and if so whether or not he might be left with some permanent disability, what effects it might have on life plans both immediate and long-range, and the special psychological meanings the illness may have for the patient, all influence his reactions to it.[6] That the feeling of danger may greatly outweigh the reality is well demonstrated by the public's reaction, for instance, to poliomyelitis. The incidence of polio is far less than that of many other even more disabling illnesses, but the fear of death or crippling give it special significance.

PSYCHOLOGY OF ANXIETY

In order to understand how anxiety develops it might be well to examine a traumatic neurosis. When an individual has a very traumatic experience, such as those encountered by many of our soldiers during the last war, he first experiences a feeling of anxiety and helplessness. This may be transient or of long duration. Usually the first reaction is to repress the memory along with the feelings and thoughts associated with the traumatic event. The individual, in other words, tries to "forget" the experience. And even though he may consciously seem to do so, the memory is not really forgotten but buried, as it were, in the unconscious area of his mind. A next step is the avoidance of all situations and actions that might possibly remind the individual of the traumatic event and thus recall it and its associated painful feelings to mind. In order to accomplish this the individual may impose many restrictions on himself. The most flagrant example of such a chain of events is seen in a case of amnesia following a traumatic experience. It may be necessary not only to forget the event but also even one's own identity, lest the recollection of who one is might carry with it the painful memory of what one has experienced.

But this effort to repress or keep out of consciousness the painful event is always in danger of failing. The feeling associated with the event may become manifest even though the event still remains repressed. The individual may feel anxious or may feel guilty or have some other unpleasant feeling without knowing why. He may even seek to minimize these feelings, through various apparently irrational forms of behavior. He may actually seek punishment for the guilt feelings, even though the reason for them is not conscious.

If his ordinary methods of defense do not succeed in keeping the painful memory from threatening to return to consciousness, the individual then may utilize modes of dealing with his problem which were characteristic of an earlier phase of his emotional development. This is the phenomenon known as regression. Ultimately the anxiety may become bound in a symptom which simultaneously expresses and conceals the conflict. These symptoms may take a tremendous variety of forms depending on the nature of the traumatic experience, the conflict it arouses and the previous history of the individual. Very often, as indicated before, the patient may complain of physical symptoms which are either the physiologic concomitants of anxiety or the symbolic expressions of the emotional conflict from which the individual is suffering. Thus in the traumatic combat neuroses we saw not only cases of amnesia already referred to, but also many other varieties of symptoms. Many soldiers became very depressed, suffered from intense feelings of guilt when, for instance, a buddy of theirs was killed on a mission with which they had nothing to do. In some instances the only connection might have been that the buddy had borrowed some garment that belonged to the surviving soldier and he feels that somehow or other he had brought his buddy bad luck. In working with such a patient, it was often not at all difficult to discover that the relationship between him and the dead buddy contained not only the more obvious element of affection but also some hostility. There was some rivalry, jealousy, or very often the relationship to the buddy was a repetition of the relationship that the patient had to his own brother with its attendant sibling rivalry.[4]

Sometimes these disturbances gave rise to somatic complaints which served not only to expiate guilt feelings through actual suffering but also to avoid return to the danger of a repetition of the traumatic experience. Although these soldiers were unable to recall the traumatic events that had precipitated their illnesses the fact that such events still had dynamic force was revealed frequently by the nightmares from which the soldiers suffered, or when under the influence of sodium amytal the whole event was not only recalled but re-experienced. A slogan we came to use in working with such patients was "the best way to forget is to remember." By bringing the experience back into consciousness, helping the patient face it along with the conflicting emotions, it was then possible for him to work it through and overcome the symptoms from which he was suffering.

EMOTIONAL DEVELOPMENT AND ANXIETY

We can now review briefly some of the main highlights of the emotional development of people in order to notice what types of anxiety occur at different stages of development and how these are defended against and, in turn, how the persistence of certain unresolved conflicts may reappear in the illnesses of adults. The newborn infant is virtually helpless; he has very intense instinctual needs and drives that must be met by the mother. When an infant is hungry or disturbed in any other way his immediate reaction is to cry, and observation of the infant readily reveals the fact that he is anxious. This cry serves the purpose of bringing the mother to the child and having her relieve the tension. The child quickly comes to recognize the mother as the object who relieves his tension and as long as she is present he does not feel helpless, but when she is absent he may become apprehensive. If the mother is sufficiently available the child soon develops a feeling of security and thus he is able to develop gradually the capacity to tolerate some tension before requiring its relief. Thus it may be said that the child actually is able to anticipate the mother's arrival even before she is physically present. If, on the other hand, the mother's care of the child is deficient the child is unable to develop the same feeling of security and therefore is apt to be tense and anxious most of the time, being unable to anticipate if and when his discomfort will be relieved. Everyone is familiar with the fact that a frightened child clings to his mother's skirt and may become very disturbed when the mother goes away despite reassurances of her return. Even children when they grow older, if they are upset by anything such as an illness may at times react in this way.

For the little weak and helpless child there are many real external dangers. In addition parents give frequent warnings against the dangers of fire, knives, streets, etc., which may tend to increase the child's feeling that without the protection of his parents he is helpless and at the mercy of a dangerous world. When instinctual tension manifests itself in the child and when the environment in the form of the mother or nurse meets the demand with indifference, with refusal, with annoyance, with threats or with punishment, that painful state has to find some other release. The child may have to suffer loneliness, hunger or whatever other discomfort he may be experiencing, and it has been observed that if he must endure tension too long he is likely to become apathetic or emotionally cold. Thus it may be that the child begins to experience not only the outside world as dangerous and painful but also may look upon his instinctual impulses as similarly dangerous or painful.

The most primitive and initial form of anxiety, therefore, is experienced when instinctual needs are not appropriately gratified and the feeling of helplessness is one of the most basic feelings that can lead to anxiety.

Gradually as the child grows older he is called upon to assume more responsibility for himself and to modify his primitive instinctual behavior in terms of the demands of society. He is taught to control his sphincters, to eat his food properly, he is called upon to keep his primitive aggression under control, to limit his curiosity and, in general, to begin to behave as a cultured civilized human being. It is primarily only because of the wish to please his parents, not to lose their love, and the associated security that the child makes efforts to comply with parental demands. Thus it is possible that some of his instinctual impulses, the direct expression of which has been prohibited or punished, may become sources of danger, for they demand expression on the one hand but lead to difficulty with significant persons in the child's life on the other hand. It is of course essential that every child be helped to modify his instinctual expressions in accordance with reality and the requirements of society. But it is preferable that the child be helped to find acceptable substitute gratifications rather than be given the feeling that he is bad, unworthy or naughty, because he feels anger or wants to play with his feces or do many other things that seem to him quite normal and in fact fun. Gradually the child incorporates within his own personality the rules of his parents and the society in which he lives. This is much more happily accomplished if he gives up some of his modes of expression because he wants to retain the parents' love, rather than out of fear of their punishment and is even more happily achieved if he is helped to find acceptable substitutes for the expression of his feelings and gratification of his needs than being called upon to restrain them completely.

As the child develops further he begins to experience erotic feelings in the area of his own genitals and also great curiosity about the sexual activity of his parents. This may also correspond to curiosity about where babies come from. Unfortunately, our culture maintains a conspiracy of silence about such interests. In his normal investigations and explorations the child will discover that playing with certain parts of his body can produce pleasurable sensations and he is likely to enjoy these without any feeling that this pleasure is any different than other pleasures except that perhaps it is greater than previous ones. However, when the parents discover that he is so engaging himself the strictest taboos, prohibitions and punishments suddenly may become imposed. The child can only be bewildered by this experience for he can see no reason why his curiosity about why some people have penises and others don't, about where babies come from, is any less acceptable than his curiosity about why the sky is blue or why it gets dark at night. He has perhaps not only been permitted but encouraged to enjoy physical sensations by being rocked, by riding on merry-go-rounds and swinging in swings but also by the pleasure of a warm bath and by being embraced by his mother. It is hard then for him to understand why the even more exciting pleasure of touching his genitals is so taboo. He can only in his immature way draw many erroneous conclusions, not the least frequent of which is that he is a naughty, bad, dirty person. Again great conflict is stimulated because of the intensity of his feelings and the barriers erected against their expression.

Like the soldier with the traumatic neurosis, the child deals with these problems by repression of the experiences and the gradual development of symptoms which will help him avoid their return to consciousness. Everyone is familiar with the childhood fears of falling, of the dark, of dying, of ghosts, of being alone, of insects, bogiemen, etc. These phobias of childhood are actually, in a sense of the word, normal, for they are almost universal in their occurrence and tend to disappear in time.

In summary, society through the parents imposes certain restrictions on the expression of instinctual impulses. For each individual the way in which these conflicts arise and are dealt with varies. But the general patterns for all people are much the same. The instinctual impulses with which we all have to learn to deal are universal and the necessity for modification of them is also experienced by everyone. However, there are great variations in regard to how parents deal with these; which are permitted greater or lesser expression, which become associated with certain life experiences, etc. No matter what the specific original event was that resulted in a conflict, as long as the conflict remains unresolved it will tend to become stimulated by subsequent life experiences which for one reason or another resemble the original experience. For instance, a child may have had to repress and deny his envy and jealousy of a more favored sibling and has attempted to do this by utilizing the mechanism of reaction formation, that is, exaggerating his affection and repressing his hostility. If he becomes attached to someone of his own approximate age later in life, he may then be prone to intense feelings of guilt if something should happen to that individual, such as in the example given before of the death of a buddy in wartime. Concealed in the close relationship may be the hostility that was originally felt toward the sibling, and the death of the buddy actually may represent the fulfillment of a repressed death wish which results in intense guilt feelings.

If a child has been frightened into giving up masturbatory impulses by being threatened with having his penis cut off, it is not at all surprising to find him experiencing intense anxiety when confronted with a simple surgical procedure such as a tonsillectomy, or when experiencing strong sexual urges.

There are many possible types of anxiety experienced in childhood which may reoccur under certain circumstances later in life. These may be separation anxiety when there is danger of the loss of a person on whom one is dependent for love and security, or may be anxiety associated with fear of punishment for giving expression to instinctual impulses which have been forbidden. There may be anxieties associated with sexual activity which is viewed as forbidden, even though the sanction of marriage removes the taboos.[1]

Thus it is possible to readily understand that there is a great variety of life experiences which can give rise to anxiety because they resemble earlier conflictual life experiences that were encountered by the individual when his ego was weak and undeveloped. If there were a great number of childhood conflicts which have remained unresolved, the ego is greatly burdened and is more vulnerable to develop anxiety than if the child's experience has been more fortunate and he has helped to learn to channelize his instinctual impulses into appropriate directions and obtain gratification through satisfactory substitute activities.

It is for these reasons that it is believed that reality experiences which precipitate anxiety are actually not the causes of the anxiety but are experiences which by association revive old conflicts. These conflicts may be stimulated either by experiences which seem to represent the punishment for forbidden activity or experiences which increase the intensity of the instinctual impulses. In many phobias one can see both mechanisms operating simultaneously. The individual fears a particular thing not only because of the punishment but also because of the temptation and like the phobias of childhood that which he fears is really a symbolic representative of some unconscious conflict.

When an individual suffers from an anxiety attack the most normal reaction is to make some aggressive effort to remove the frustration and conflict. On the one hand he may attempt to obtain gratification despite the cost; on the other hand he may achieve a mature solution which allows acceptable gratification and retention of the love of the love object whose loss he may have feared. If unable to solve his problem in these ways he may regress and develop a neurosis. Actually all neuroses start with an anxiety attack of some sort.[3]

MAKING A DIAGNOSIS

In order to treat the anxious patient it is as imperative to make an accurate diagnosis as it is in trying to treat any other medical problem. One must always do an adequate physical examination in order carefully to rule out organic disease. It is very tempting to dismiss obscure physical complaints as neurotic without thorough physical investigation especially with patients who have been previously known to be prone to neurotic reactions. However, the diagnosis of a psychiatric disturbance should not be made by exclusion alone, nor should it be made because of the failure of various attempts through medical therapy to relieve the patient of his symptoms. Such pseudo-diagnostic methods not only reflect poor medical practice but also may tend to fix the idea of organic disease in the patient's mind. In making a psychiatric diagnosis attaching the appropriate diagnostic label to the patient's illness is of minimal usefulness. It is necessary to have an understanding of what it is the patient is reacting to at the time and in what way he is reacting (the dynamic diagnosis), as well as to understand something of the life history of the patient and its relation to the current problem (genetic diagnosis).[2]

TREATMENT

Following such an appraisal of the patient's problem the physician is in a position to estimate the treatment goals and to ascertain whether or not he is professionally equipped to treat the patient or should refer him to a psychiatrist.

If the anxiety attack is in any way related to an actual physical illness, the physical illness must, of course, be properly treated. However, as far as anxiety itself is concerned, it should be evident from what already has been said that the ideal treatment goal would be that of helping the patient become conscious of the nature of the inner conflict which has become stimulated by the reality situation which precipitated the illness and helping him, on the one hand, to resolve the conflict and, on the other hand, to find acceptable means of gratification. It is a great temptation to utilize the various sedatives as a means of helping the individual allay his anxiety. While these may have very great value for the relief of the symptom, they are obviously useless as a cure. To depend entirely on the use of sedatives is to actually postpone the appropriate treatment and thus may not only help fix the idea in the mind of the patient that he is suffering from something organic but also make any subsequent psychological approach more difficult.

Another common tendency, particularly with phobic patients, is to try to get them to face their phobias. In view of the fact that the phobia is merely a substitute for what the patient is really frightened of, it is evident that this has little value. No one is really afraid of the dark, of closets, or of heights, and thus taking him into the dark or into a closet or on top of a tall building does not solve the conflict. Phobias do not respond to sensible reassurance, even when this is given by someone who is loved and trusted.

Patients generally come to physicians with a positive attitude. They have trust that the doctor is competent to help them and this in itself helps to allay some of the intensity of their anxiety feelings. They look upon the physician as someone on whom they can be legitimately dependent, as someone who will help them solve their problems, as someone who is kindly, objective, and nonjudgmental, and as someone who is both omniscient and omnipotent. In general the doctor is viewed as an ideal, benign, father figure. There are patients, however, who approach the doctor with mixed feelings. Along with the feelings of trust just mentioned may be feelings of fear that the doctor in some way will discover the patient's secrets and will punish rather than forgive. Many illnesses and surgical procedures are viewed in just this way.

The doctor's behavior tends to confirm the patient's attitudes. He first listens carefully to the patient's recitation of his problems. He is patient, and waits until he has sufficient understanding of what the patient is telling him before expressing any opinions. His opinions in turn ordinarily are objective and based primarily on his understanding of the patient's illness rather than subjective in terms of judgments.[5]

Following this hearing of the patient's history he carefully examines the patient. This is a special privilege accorded to doctors and the patient may not only uncover his body but also his feelings. Finally the physician diagnoses and prescribes, rather than condemns or punishes. Oftentimes it is sufficient for the patient to have an opportunity to talk to someone who listens to his problems in the way that a physician should regularly do. If, through his careful examinations, the doctor finds that there is no evidence of organic illness, this alone may give the patient great comfort. However, it is not sufficient to let things rest at this point, it is much better if the doctor were to go on to inquire into the patient's life in order to determine what might be distressing him and thus help him realize where his problems really lie. Many patients derive great benefit from telling their troubles to someone who is willing to listen and will be accepting. "Getting it off one's chest" is a well-known means of obtaining relief. In doing so the patient may feel much less alone than before and as a consequence may be able to achieve greater objectivity about himself and through the experience of being able to talk to someone he may become more generally spontaneous.

Oftentimes by permitting the patient to talk, the patient himself achieves some clarification and understanding of his problem. It is not uncommon to have a patient say, after he has been talking for a long period of time and the doctor has done nothing more than listen, "Thank you, doctor, you've been a great help to me." The doctor might be quite mystified or confused because he thinks he has done nothing, but by his patient listening and acceptance he has actually done a great deal.

The physician, by indicating that other people have similar problems and feelings, further decreases the sense of isolation, shame and guilt which many patients feel. "Confession is good for the soul" and it is further very reassuring to find that other people harbor similar unacceptable thoughts at times.

As the physician discusses the patient's life history with him the patient may often be led to an understanding of the connection between current events and past patterns of behavior and reactions. Patients can often acquire some intellectual insight into the relationships between situations, affects and symptoms and alter their situation and/or their response in a healthier manner. Through carefully directed questions the physician may help the patient not only achieve some understanding of his problems but also lead him spontaneously to a solution. The solution of surface conflicts can often restore peace of mind, and finding better modes of expression of one's feelings leads to greater ease.

The physician who is not trained in psychiatry should limit his attention to the patient's conscious feelings even though he may be aware of certain unconscious factors in the problem. He should also be aware that patients tend to endow him with attributes that he does not possess and have feelings of affection and anger for him that are unrelated and inappropriate to the doctor-patient relationship. The tendency of patients to look upon the doctor as a magical omnipotent father figure on whom they can become dependent and who will solve their problems for them may be very flattering. The doctor, however, must wisely avoid falling into this trap for sooner or later he will be unable to meet the patient's demands, his magic may fail to work and the affection and co-operation may turn into anger and negativism. Such transference feelings, as they are called, are echoes of early childhood relationships in the life of the patient and are part of the patient's neurotic conflict and therefore need to be recognized as symptomatic of his illness.

It also must be appreciated that although the patient is unhappy and wants help, another part of him resists giving up his symptoms. The symptom is there for a reason; it has a purpose and satisfies a certain craving of the patient's unconscious. Consequently, any effort to change it meets with opposition. This resistance to getting well may manifest itself in a great variety of ways. It may be hidden in the transference feelings of the patient, it may take the form of a "flight into health," the patient may miss his appointments, refuse to see his role in his difficulties attributing all his troubles to others, etc.

When the doctor becomes aware of the patient's resistance he may become annoyed just as he may have been flattered by the patient's docile obedience. Such countertransference reactions as these (and others) are not only inappropriate but also undesirable. The physician must at all times maintain his objectivity if he is to be truly helpful.

Since anxiety, no matter what its cause or how it may be expressed, is a symptom of emotional conflict, treatment requires understanding of the conflict. This implies understanding of the person who has the conflict. It is this understanding, first by the physician and, in turn, by the patient, which constitutes the basis of the treatment.

BIBLIOGRAPHY

1. English, O. Spurgeon, and Pearson, G. H. J.: Emotional Problems of Living, New York, Norton, 1945.
2. Levine, Maurice: Psychotherapy in Medical Practice, New York, Macmillan, 1942.
3. Menninger, K. A.: The Human Mind, New York, Knopf, 1937.
4. ———: Man Against Himself, New York, Harcourt Brace, 1938.
5. ———: A Manual for Psychiatric Case Study, New York, Grune & Stratton, 1952.
6. Coleman, Jules V.: Consider the Emotions, Bull. Nat. Tuberc. Assn. 41:157-158, 1955.

4

THE DEPRESSED PATIENT

Franklin G. Ebaugh, M.D.

". . . lean, withered, hollow-eyed, look old, wrinkled, harsh, troubled much with wind, and a griping in their bellies, or belly-ache, belch often, dry bellies and hard, dejected looks, flaggy beards, singing of the ears, vertigo, lightheaded, little or no sleep, and that interrupt, terrible and fearful dreams . . ."; thus Hippocrates described his melancholic patients, as quoted by Robert Burton in "The Anatomy of Melancholy."[1] This Latin treatise by an English clergyman, published in 1628, is a fascinating compilation of medieval and ancient thought concerning melancholic disease, wherein the psychiatrist of today may clearly recognize not only familiar combinations of physical and mental symptoms, but also many familiar attitudes toward the etiology and treatment of those disorders in which depression appears as the most significant symptom.

Among the most frequently quoted of Burton's sources, Aretaeus of Cappadocia, a practicing physician in Rome during the second century A.D., appears to have most nearly anticipated modern thought concerning depressive illness. His writings reveal an interest in the pre-morbid temperament or personality of his mentally ill patients, a sound basis of differentiation of various types of mental illness, and a widely heralded ability to state the prognosis of a particular mental illness. In addition, he indicated a recognition of the cyclic nature of depressive types of illness and recognized some connection with manic disorders.[2]

In 1854, Falret published the first modern paper recognizing this cyclic factor in many of the severely depressed patients he had studied and noted that a manic state furnished the second half of the cycle. He termed the condition so characterized *la folie circulaire*. At about the same time, Baillarger announced similar

47

observations and termed the condition *folie à double forme*. In the German psychiatric thought of this period organic factors were considered the sole cause of mental illness, and hence all emphasis was placed on classification according to pathologic and physiologic principles from which the organic pathology might be discovered. In 1862, Kahlbaum,[3] a leader of the German school, described the milder emotional cyclic changes from hypomania to mild depression and termed the condition cyclothymia. It was with the firm conviction of the organically determined nature of mental illness that Kraepelin derived and presented, in 1901, the classical classification of mental disease in which he combined the observations of the ancients, Falret, Baillarger and Kahlbaum, with his own meticulous work into the concept of the manic-depressive psychoses. Except for two depressive syndromes which he termed involutional melancholia and "psychogenic depression," Kraepelin combined all mental disorders with mania or depression as cardinal symptoms into the concept of the manic-depressive group differentiating the pure affective states and the "mixed types" within the group. A few years later, based on the work of Dreyfus, Kraepelin included the originally separate involutional melancholia in the manic-depressive concept, and discussed the pre-psychotic temperaments or "fundamental states" of manic-depressive patients, classifying them as depressive, manic, irritable or cyclothymic after Reiss.[4] Kraepelin stressed his evidence for the hereditary nature of these temperament types as well as of the manic-depressive psychoses themselves. He further pointed out the "recoverability" or self-limiting tendency of this class of mental disease, making this a major point of differentiation from the dementia praecox group.

Drawing from the concepts of Charcot, Bernheim and Janet, the developing psychoanalytic theory and treatment under Sigmund Freud initially was concerned with deriving psychological concepts of neurotic illness. In so doing, however, theories of personality development and dynamics were produced which appeared susceptible of more general application to the understanding of pathologic behavior. The first attempt at dynamic and developmental understanding of depressive illness in psychological terms was made by Abraham,[5] a co-worker of Freud's, in 1912. Abraham related the pre-morbid personality structure of depressives to early infantile disappointments with resultant ambivalent attitudes toward objects of affection and identification. During the further development of the personality these ambivalently perceived love objects have their attributes incorporated or introjected as an integral part of the infant or child's personality. Due

TABLE 1. HISTORICAL DEVELOPMENT OF CONCEPTS OF DEPRESSION

ca. 400 B.C.	Hippocrates	Description of depressive illness
ca. 200 A.D.	Aretaeus	Periodicity, relationship to mania, and prognosis
1628	Burton	Compilation of ancient and medieval concepts in "The Anatomy of Melancholy"
1854	Falret	*La folie circulaire*
1854	Baillarger	*Folie à double forme*
1862	Kahlbaum	Cyclothymia
1901	Kraepelin	Manic-depressive psychoses, organic, hereditary, cyclic, recoverable. Pre-psychotic temperament types
1912	Abraham	Initial psychodynamic (psychoanalytic) interpretation of depression as hostility toward internalized love object
1915	Freud	Psychoanalytic concept of relation of depression to normal grief, and basis of psychotherapeutic treatment
1915	Meyer, A.	Psychobiological approach and mental illness as a maladjustive reaction
1927	Kretschmer	Attempts to relate temperament and types of mental illness to anthropometric studies
1928	Rado	Relation of self-esteem and depression. Periodicity of depression related to biologic periodicity of hunger and satiation
1933	Sakel	Insulin coma treatment of psychoses
1934	Meduna	Metrazol convulsive treatment of psychoses
1936	Moniz	Original psychosurgical technics introduced
1938	Cerletti and Bini	Electroconvulsive treatment
1940-1955	Selye et al.	Endocrine and biochemical reactions to life stresses

to the disappointments and resulting ambivalence of the child, hostility toward the love object and those perceived as equivalent during later life, becomes directed inwardly against the introjected object and thus apparently against the self in self-accusation and self-deprecation. This self-punishment is further intensified by the reproaches of the patient from the internalized object with the implied threat of withdrawal of love from the patient, which in its original infantile form gained the meaning of withdrawal of the means of survival. Freud, in 1915, further developed the psychoanalytic interpretation in a comparison of normal mourning over the death of a love object and the internal loss of love of an introjected love object.[6] The most recent major contribution to the psychoanalytic interpretation of depression was made by Rado in 1928,[7] when he further interpreted the self-reproaches of the depressed patient as attempts at ingratiation of the introjected, ambivalently perceived love-object. He indicates the importance of self-esteem in the depressed patient and the effective destruction of it by the psychodynamics of depression. Rado also implies, in this early paper, a denial of depression through utilization of euphoria or mania and indicates a possible basis of periodicity of manic-depressive disorders in the hunger-satiety pattern of the infant. In a later paper,[8] Rado goes beyond previous dynamic formulations to a discussion of hedonic control mechanisms and their importance in the rational planning of therapy in the depressive disorders.

Freud, Abraham and Rado, as well as other psychoanalytic writers, have indicated the occurrence of constitutional predisposing factors in the development of depression in some if not all patients. Because their principal concern was elucidation of psychodynamics of mental disease, this constitutional factor is often lost sight of in discussion of their concepts. It emerges, however, when explanation is sought for the variation in depressive syndromes. Three main considerations appear to account for this variation: (1) the strength of constitutional factors (e.g., constitutional tendency to oral eroticism), (2) degree of infantile disappointment and deprivation, and (3) severity of originally external suppressive measures directed against the expression of hostility by the infant or child. A fourth consideration may be the degree of obvious and conscious similarity of the adult situation and social relationships at the time of the illness, to the early emotional experiences which may be recapitulated in the unconscious feeling of the patient.

Meyer and his co-workers have influenced the general thoughts regarding mental illness by their emphasis on the typical patterns of reaction to life situations which a given individual builds from his intimately combined organic endowment and his experience. Mental illness is then perceived as a reaction to stress situations by application of faulty or inappropriate habit patterns typical for the individual as a psychobiological unit. Present diagnostic terminology reflects this concept in the designation of disease entities as reactions. Under Meyer's influence there also developed the concept of "affective disorders," thus improving understanding of the symptomatic relationship of this class of disorder to mental illness as a whole. Perhaps most important, Meyer's conceptual position is increasingly proving its adaptability as a meeting place for divergent views on the relative importance of organic and psychodynamic factors in mental illness.

Working from Kraepelin's concepts, Kretschmer, in 1927, published the results of his attempt to correlate temperament and types of mental illness with factors of body build. He reported that two-thirds of manic-depressive patients exhibited a *pyknic,* or short, stout physique.[9] A failure to find rigid, objective standards for evaluating body build made duplication of Kretschmer's work difficult for other workers. However, in 1940, Sheldon published a rigid, objective system of body measurement which he termed somatotyping, and reported a high correlation between certain somatotypes and personality types.[10] Sheldon's work received support from several other investigators, but serious, as yet unanswered questions were raised by the work of Lasker[11] who demonstrated definite and significant changes in somatotypes with changes in dietary habits.

Into a short five years were crowded the major developments in the so-called somatic therapies of mental illness. In 1933, M. Sakel introduced insulin coma therapy of psychotic illness; the following year, Meduna began the use of metrazol for the induction of convulsion as a treatment of schizophrenia; and in 1936, Moniz performed surgery on the frontal portion of the brain of a psychotic patient and reported improvement in the chronic mental illness. Probably the most significant development for the treatment of the affective disorders came as a result of the search for a technic which avoided the undesirable side-effects of Meduna's metrazol while retaining its apparently beneficial convulsive action. Cerletti and Bini reported such a technic in electroconvulsive treatments in 1938. The effects of these discoveries on the treatment of affective disorders will be discussed in another context.

From ancient periods when an excess of black bile was considered etiologically significant in cases of depression, there have been numerous theories involving endocrine, autonomic and central nervous system dysfunction in the etiology of depression and other mental disorders without currently demonstrable organic pathology. Many investigations have been directed toward definition of variations in the biochemical and neurologic function of mental patients and their deviations from the normal population. While much of this work has to date been inconclusive and contradictions are frequent, there can be no doubt that whatever the psychodynamics of a given reaction, that reaction takes place on and is mediated by a physiologic, biochemical, organic substrate. Any possibility of rapidly altering the course of mental illness would appear to be based on the possibility of effecting controlled changes, by drugs or other means, in the organic substrate rather than by the arduous and delicate technics directed at psychologic re-integration and corrective experience. Certainly such psychotherapeutic and re-educative technics must also be employed in most cases for stabilization and adjustment to life situations either disrupted by the illness or contributing to the illness. It is therefore understandable that biologic research in mental illness has received great impetus from the work of Selye and his formulation of physiologic responses as adaptive attempts of the organism to various types of stress. Physiologic and biochemical concomitants of the depressive syndromes will be further discussed with symptomatology.

Two classifications of the depressive disorders are presented in Table 2. The first, and most elaborate, is William A. White's modification of Kraepelin's original classification with its division into subtypes and mixed types.[12] The second classification is that adopted by the American Psychiatric Association in 1952.

Kraepelin and many others considered all of the depressive reactions other than the specific, neurotic, psychogenic depression to be endogenous and unrelated to situational factors. As indicated by Bellak,[13] there is some justification for conceiving a continuum of depressive reactions from a hypothetically completely organic determination to a hypothetically completely experiential determination. He further suggests, based on Freud's concept of symptoms as compromise formation, that a continuum according to ego strength extends from hypothetical "normalcy" to schizophrenic deterioration, through the intermediate points of neurotic and manic-depressive disorders. According to his concepts these two continua are independent in such manner that full understanding of an individual patient's disorder would ideally require

TABLE 2. CLASSIFICATIONS OF DEPRESSIVE DISORDERS

Kraepelin (Modif. White)	A.P.A. (1952)
Manic-Depressive Psychoses	Manic-depressive reaction,
Depressive phase	depressive type
Simple retardation	Manic-depressive reaction,
Acute melancholia	other (specify)
Depressive stupor	Psychotic depressive reaction
Periodical psychoses	
Recurrent melancholia	
Alternating insanity	Involutional depressive reaction
Circular insanity	
Mixed states	
Maniacal stupor	Schizophrenic reaction,
Agitated depression	schizo-affective type
Unproductive mania	
Depressive mania	
Depression with flight of ideas	
Akinetic mania	
Involutional Melancholia	
Psychogenic Depression	Depressive reaction (neurotic)

this assignment to a relative position on each scale. Unfortunately, this can rarely be done with the present technics and with present knowledge, but the recent A.P.A. classification of depressive syndromes, in Table 2, tends toward the recognition of this frame of reference.

Depressive reactions, corresponding to Kraepelin's psychogenic depression, are generally agreed to be predominantly determined by environmental factors and the neurotic reactions of the patient. In these reactive depressions, according to the analytic view, the patient attempts to force from the environment those needed emotional satisfactions which have been inadequate or absent. This aggressive attitude produces guilt and fear of retaliation by the environment and hence those inward feelings which the patient recognizes as a depressed mood. Unlike the psychotic depressive, these patients recognize their discomfort is a reaction to some environmental factor, and they clearly distinguish that which is within them and that which is external. Anxiety symptoms may be present in these patients but are secondary in importance to the depressive affect, lack of concentration, and general loss of interest. Loss of self-esteem in some failure is frequently a precipitating factor in reactive depression, but as noted by Fenichel,[14] success may be a precipitating factor if such success is seen as a threat of further demands, or as occasion for jealous aggression from the environment in retaliation. Brief psychotherapy of a supporting and mildly interpretive type is usually adequate treatment in these reactions.

Fenichel indicates the manner in which the relatively mild reactive depression may progress to the more severe psychotic depressive reaction (A.P.A.) through the sequence "You don't satisfy me—I hate you"; "You don't satisfy me—I hate me"; "I don't satisfy myself—I hate myself," as a result of more intense hostility or less satisfactory environment. Where the ego or personality development has been weakened by early experiences of this type, regression to earlier developmental levels occurs in the patient and clear differentiation between self and environment becomes difficult or impossible. Suicidal preoccupation, self-depreciation and self-punishment become prominent features. Patients of this type may be troubled with the same somatic complaints, retardation, perceptive distortions, and delusions as the manic-depressive reaction, depressed type discussed below, and essentially the same treatment principles govern both. The classical Kraepelinian classification makes no distinction between the groups.

As previously mentioned, Kraepelin came to consider that involutional melancholy was only a manic-depressive psychosis occurring at climacteric, a view that has not gained wide acceptance. Henderson and Gillespie[15] state that their experience indicates involutional melancholia to be a relatively common type of mental disorder with certain definite features of its own, namely, depression without retardation, anxiety, a feeling of unreality, and hypochondriacal or nihilistic delusions. The occurrence of this combination of symptoms in the involutional period, without prior history of mental illness, is felt to justify the diagnosis of involutional melancholia. Strecker, Ebaugh and Ewalt[16] stress the importance of the depressive-apprehensive affect in this class of patient and indicate the frequency of agitation and negativism resembling that encountered in catatonic patients. Physical symptoms are variable but generally similar to those of other severe depressions with anorexia, insomnia and constipation being most frequent. Henderson and Gillespie, Noyes,[17] and others comment on the marked differences in pre-psychotic personalities of the typical involutional melancholic contrasted with the typical manic-depressive patient. While the manic-depressive patient has typically shown considerable affective swings (cyclothymic) and tends to be aggressively optimistic or pessimistic, the involutional melancholic typically has been overconscientious, shy, rigid and sensitive. Etiologically, the organic substrate plays a more obvious role in this class of disorder than in the two previously discussed categories, but most present-day psychiatrists consider that the involutional changes with resultant increased irritability of the autonomic nervous system are not primary in the affective disorder, but rather the patient's reaction to perceived changes and the loss of prized functions threatens an already insecure personality which may have previously been defended by reaction-formations against strong aggressive impulses. Treatment principles are similar to those for the manic-depressive depressions insofar as the acute illness is concerned. Electroconvulsive treatments appear particularly efficacious in this group, and with proper precautions, organic contraindications are rare. Psychotherapeutic follow-up in these cases is almost exclusively supportive and directed at broadening of interests as well as maintenance of good physical hygiene.

The three previously discussed depressive groups, with the manic-depressive depressions, may be recognized to include all the combinations of organic and psychodynamic etiologic factors, but in terms of personality deterioration the extreme of deterioration is not reached in any of the affective reactions. When this extreme is reached in other than a severe organic condition, a diagnosis of schizophrenia is usually made. Frequently differential diagnosis between manic-depressive reactions and schizophrenic reactions is extremely difficult since, as Noyes comments, "—just as personalities are not cast in standardized molds so we find all gradations between those reactions we call schizophrenic and those we call manic-depressive." The present A.P.A. classification takes this into account and bridges the gap with the diagnostic group schizophrenic reaction, schizo-affective type.

Manic-depressive reaction, depressive type, and manic-depressive reaction, other (specify) of the A.P.A. classification include all of the depressive and mixed depressive variations in which the depression is felt to be endogenous and appears unrelated to environmental factors. Constitutional and hereditary factors are widely felt to be primary as etiologic agents, and periodicity, either in terms of recurrent affective reactions or of pre-morbid tendencies to cyclic affective swings, is considered as an outstanding characteristic. Many psychoanalytic writers feel that even within this classification there exist vast differences in the relative importance of organic and infantile environmental factors. Their views in this matter have been discussed previously, but it should be added that, in the opinion of many, the existence of strong constitutional factors in a given patient does not preclude the existence of typical psychodynamic patterns, an understanding of which may be of inestimable value to the management of the patient in his life situation.

Numerous studies have been made toward the establishment of the importance of hereditary factors in manic-depressive disease and have, in the majority of instances, produced statistical evidence supporting the assumption of constitutional predisposition. Most convincing of these studies are those of Slater[18] and Kallmann[19] on the manic-depressive expectancy rates of the parents and siblings of monozygotic and dizygotic twins with manic depressive disease. Kallmann reports on a series of 27 monozygotic and 55 dizygotic manic-depressive twins and finds an expectancy rate of 16.7 per cent for half-siblings, 22.7 per cent for full siblings, 25.5 per cent for dizygotic co-twins, and 100 per cent for monozygotic co-twins, and compared with a maximum expectancy of 0.4 per cent for the general population. Slater's findings, on somewhat smaller group, are exactly parallel. It would be very difficult to explain the above figures purely on the basis of the similar environmental and psychodynamic factors in a given family, but Kallmann comments, "The dynamics identified with this specific (genetic) ability cannot be considered to be part of person's normal biological equipment nor are they out of line with current concepts of psychodynamic phenomena as observed in potentially vulnerable persons."

Attempts at division of depressive disease into numerous sub-classifications, according to symptomatic minutia on the part of Kraepelin and others, are regarded by most psychiatrists as not clinically useful since such symptoms will vary with the previous personality and experience of the individual patient. Therefore, current discussion is usually in terms of the severity of the depression, varying from simple retardation (mild depression, simple depression) to acute depression (severe depression), and depressive

TABLE 3.   SPONTANEOUS COMPLAINTS OF DEPRESSED PATIENTS

Psychic Complaints:	Physical Complaints:
Lack of interest	Weakness
Impaired concentration	Headache, often ill-defined and ill-localized
Sense of being slowed in thought and action	Indigestion, epigastric distress and distention
Sense of inadequacy and loss of confidence	Chronic fatigue
Indecisiveness	Loss of sexual desire and potency
A "lost" feeling	Weight loss
Preoccupation with fears and doubts	
Feelings of unworthiness and guilt	

stupor. Agitation in a depressive illness is considered merely as symptomatic evidence of greater anxiety in the individual patient. Alternating states, however, offer additional problems in terms of psychodynamics, as previously mentioned.

Depression or depressive mood per se is a spontaneous complaint in only a minority of manic-depressive, depressed patients, and even on interrogation such feelings may be denied or recognized only as a mild downheartedness. Symptoms generally are predominately mental or predominately physical and may be exclusively physical. Campbell finds that physical complaints related to autonomic nervous system dysfunction are much more frequent than are the mental complaints and points out the frequency of various physical diagnoses in these patients.[20] In Table 3 are listed the complaints which seem to be most frequently given by the depressed patient spontaneously. Usually only three or four complaints are volunteered and not infrequently a single physical symptom may be the only spontaneous complaint. In those cases of severe depression (acute depression or depressive stupor) there may, of course, be no spontaneous complaints at all or only self-accusatory statements and protestations of unworthiness and hopelessness. Table 4 lists those complaints frequently revealed by questioning the depressed patient, though these complaints may of course be given spontaneously.

Many of the complaints of depressed patients will be given a delusional quality by the manner of their expression, but as with the hallucinations, which may also be present, they appear as an overemphasis on certain aspects of reality and a misinterpretation under the influence of a dominant affect rather than a bizarre

TABLE 4.   COMPLAINTS REVEALED ON QUESTIONING DEPRESSED PATIENTS

Psychic Complaints:	Physical Complaints:
"Blue spells"	Anorexia
Chronic worrying	Poor sleep and early awakening
Anxiety	Constipation
Irritability	Diminution or cessation of menses
Hopelessness	
Inexplicability of illness	
Depressive mood	

reconstruction and distortion of reality as seen in a schizophrenic reaction.

Many features of differential diagnosis from the schizophrenic reactions have been previously mentioned or implied, but the frequency of change of diagnosis from manic-depressive reaction, to schizophrenic reaction testifies to the difficulty of such differentiation in early stages. A set of criteria of reported value in this matter was recently offered by Lewis and Piotrowski.[21] These authors list ten signs: (1) Physical sensation with dissociation; (2) delusions regarding others; (3) delusions regarding physical objects; (4) feeling of physical isolation and personal unreality; (5) inability to concentrate; (6) speech disturbance and intellectual blocking; (7) feeling of having changed; (8) uncontrolled repeated interrupting, and anxious thoughts (hallucinations); (9) ideas of reference and/or feeling of being controlled by inimical outside forces (paranoid ideas); and (10) seclusiveness maintained or increased in the hospital. Lewis applied these criteria to 62 patients who proved to be schizophrenic after originally being diagnosed either as manic-depressive, depressed or psychoneurotic, and also to 32 patients who proved to be manic-depressive, depressed, after long observation. It was found that the proven manic-depressive group showed an average of 0.30 of these signs per patient while the total schizophrenic group showed an average of 3.37 per patient. Signs 5 and 9 were least reliable in that they were each present in four of the manic-depressive group.

Particularly in the older age group of depressive patients, care must be taken to detect signs of organic brain damage due to the relatively rare types of degenerative brain disease, syphilis, or arteriosclerotic changes. Careful physical and laboratory examination will usually eliminate these possibilities. Careful physical

TABLE 5. COMMON FINDINGS ON PHYSICAL AND LABORATORY EXAMINATION OF DEPRESSED PATIENTS

Physical:	Laboratory:
Retardation of speech, thought and action	Defective sugar tolerance
Poor hydration and nutrition	Psychological Tests:
Sad, apprehensive facies	Higher verbal than performance
Slowed pulse rate and decreased blood pressure (variable)	Affective coloring on projection

examination has additional importance in enabling the physician to be more sincere in his reassurance to the patient, and it must be kept in mind that the presence of mental illness is no guarantee against concomitant physical illness.

In Table 5 are listed the more common physical and laboratory findings in the depressed patient. These findings are of course dependent on the severity of the depression and the duration prior to examination, and are in the most part general findings of poor nutritional status and a low level of physiologic activity.

Hundreds of studies have been made of the biochemical and endocrine concomitants of manic-depressive depressions, but consistent findings are extremely rare. Most consistent has been the finding of defective sugar tolerance confirmed by nearly all investigators.[22] Other findings reported with some consistency are increased blood levels of calcium and cholesterol. Endocrine studies have been generally contradictory; however, the work of Selye and the observed effects of ACTH on affect have spurred this type of investigation. One of the most promising of the recent studies is that of Reiss who reports that while no significant correlation can be found between the function of any one gland and a depressive state, it is established, in many of the patients investigated, there was an abnormal thyroid-adrenal cortex equilibrium which improved parallel with the improvement of the mental state.[23] This finding supports the endocrine equilibrium theories and investigations of Sackler, et al.[24]

Psychometric examinations are often very helpful in the differential diagnosis of depression. Typically the depressed patient will show a sharp superiority of verbal I.Q. over performance I.Q., reflecting in the various tests the retention of previously learned material as against the loss of ability to perform rapidly in new

TABLE 6.   PRECIPITATING FACTORS OF MANIC-DEPRESSIVE REACTIONS

Death, illness, or peril of a significant person (family member, or close companion).

Economic difficulties or threat of loss of economic security.

Marital maladjustments (infidelity, failure of emotional satisfaction, physical abuse).

Physical condition (personal illness or handicap, pregnancy, surgery, accident).

Social disapproval, present or threatened.

Personal failures of attainment or self-realization.

Jealousy and hostility (unconscious) over attainment of significant competitors.

Apparent hostility or slights from significant individuals (parents, siblings, children, close companions).

---

situations. Variability with the various sub-tests is considerably less than that seen in early schizophrenic illness. The Rorschach protocols of depressed individuals usually show an absence of, or marked reduction of, both color responses and human movement responses. While responses of a gloomy type regarding rotting, dried, old and deteriorating objects are very frequent, these responses lack the bizarre, violent, autistic and often nauseating quality typical of schizophrenia. High quality form perception, animal responses in the majority, and a small number of whole responses are other depressive indicators. Klopfer and Kelley[25] differentiate manic-depressive depressions from other types on the basis of the approximate equality of human movement responses and the sum of color responses in the manic-depressive types contrasted with a larger number of movement responses in the other types. As would be predicted, Thematic Apperception Test studies indicate a relative sterility of productions, most of which reflect a pessimistic outlook, particularly as to final outcome. Some reports indicate the presence of this type of material is also found in the majority of manic-depressive, manic type.

Although, as previously stated, manic-depressive depressions are usually characterized by relatively less obvious environmental

TABLE 7. PSYCHODYNAMICS OF DEPRESSION

Infantile Experiences:	Subsequent Recapitulation:
Complete dependence on mother figure for all satisfaction and life.	Continued strong feelings of unsatisfied dependency (unconscious).
Partial deprivation or dissatisfaction and disappointment with mother figure.	Circumstantial blow to confidence in independent ability to satisfy needs (conscious).
Hostility toward mother figure, overt.	Dissatisfaction with supplies from the environment and resultant hostility repressed.
Overt hostility met with counter-hostility.	Perception of similarities to infantile experience (unconscious).
Repression of hostility and ingratiation attempts.	Present environment emotionally equated with internalized parental images (unconscious).
Crystallization of this pattern of managing hostility.	Present increased dependency demands and hostility add to and reawaken original internalized conflict.
Identification with and internalization of parental figures (super-ego or conscience).	
Turning of hostility against internalized parent image.	
Hostile reproaches from internalized parent image (internalized counter-hostility.	

determinants, it is the widespread clinical impression that in at least four-fifths of patients with this condition precipitating factors with definite temporal and psychodynamic relationship to the onset of the illness may be determined. As might be anticipated, clinical observation reveals a rough inverse relationship between the predisposition severity, either psychodynamic or organic or combination of both, and the severity of environmental and life stresses identifiable as precipitating factors in the illness of an individual patient. Several authors have offered classifications of precipitating factors observed in manic-depressive depression. Table 6 lists a number of these environmental factors.[26, 27, 28]

Brief consideration of those factors listed in Table 6 reveals the pre-eminence of three interrelated types of present or threatened factors: (1) loss of confidence by the individual in his own ability to supply his own needs; (2) reduction of supplies from the envi-

TABLE 8.　GENERAL PRINCIPLES OF THERAPY OF DEPRESSION

Protection of Patient (hospitalization or special nursing):
　　From suicide.
　　From imprudent social and financial action under the influence of feelings of desperation or hopelessness.
　　From imprudent and mistaken attempts of friends and relatives to cajole, humor, shame or force the patient "out of it."
Improvement of Physical Status (physiotherapy, drugs and nursing):
　　By correction of sleep disturbance.
　　By careful attention to nutrition.
　　By correction of constipation.
Relief of Depressive Affect (mild psychotherapy, somatic therapy):
　　With reassurance as to prognosis and mild interpretations of the general nature of the disease.
　　With demonstrated interest in the patient and acceptance of both dependence and hostility.
　　With distracting, undemanding occupation.
　　With suitable somatic therapy.
　　With mild stimulant drugs (?).
Stabilization of Gains and Prevention of Rut-Formation (re-educative and ventilating psychotherapy, occupational therapy and social work):
　　Slowly progressive revelation of patient's patterns of handling hostility and dependency needs.
　　Examination, with the patient, of precipitating or aggravating environmental situations and their possible modifications.
　　Encouragement toward increased activity and interests.
　　Gradual re-introduction of normal responsibilities.
　　Social work contact with family to increase their understanding and co-operation toward manipulation or modification of precipitating or aggravating environmental factors.

ronment and from particular individuals; and (3) increased provocation of hostility in the individual toward the very environmental sources of supply on which he is most dependent. This of course is a restatement of the basic psychodynamic pattern previously discussed and now summarized in Table 7 as a basis for discussion of one of the aspects of treatment and management of manic-depressive depressed patients.

In the milder depressions psychotherapeutic technics alone may be adequate for treatment and management; however, in the majority of manic-depressive reactions immediate psychotherapeutic management is inadequate, impractical and inadvisable. Psychotherapy generally requires a degree of co-operation and participation by the patient which is impossible for the more severely depressed patient, even if the patient was interested in or hopeful about such therapeutic attempts. Table 8 outlines the general principles of treatment of these patients.

Suicide is the leading cause of death in psychiatric patients, excluding the oldest age groups, and is the most serious complication of depressive disease. Many physicians consider every depressed patient potentially suicidal and, it must be admitted, there are no criteria for the estimation of suicidal risk which even approach infallibility. Many mild depressions, however, may best respond to re-education and environmental manipulation which affords minimal interruption to the normal and necessary activities of the patient. In such cases, as Diethelm[29] and others have suggested, the risk involved should be carefully impressed upon the relatives with insistence that they share in the responsibility. Too, the physician must be in a position to have frequent contact with his patient sufficient to make very frequent re-evaluations of suicidal potential. Only under the most favorable and unusual circumstances should a more severely depressed patient be treated outside a hospital setting. Among the most prominent suicidal indicators are: (1) suicidal preoccupation and talk; (2) severe hypochondriasis; (3) ideas of guilt, self-deprecation, and self-accusation associated with tension and agitation; (4) feelings of futility and hopelessness; (5) severe concern about insomnia; and, (6) previous suicidal attempts.[30] Presence of these findings in obvious degree should warn the physician of high suicidal potential and should probably require close precautionary control in a suitable hospital. It has been commonly observed that depressed patients may show a definite improvement just prior to suicide, and frequently those responsible for their care have been thus deceived into relaxation of precautions. This same relaxation may occur at one of the two most dangerous periods in the treatment of depressives, namely, at the beginning of improvement in the general condition of the patient, when tragedy may be the result of an improperly trained staff and inadequate contact between physician and staff. Such results are less frequent during the other danger period when the patient is relatively early in his illness and not yet to the full depths of his illness, since at that time the physician's warning is still fresh and the staff alert.

But the risk of suicide is not always the only protective reason for hospitalizing a depressed patient. Not infrequently the patient is subjected to a variety of attempts to cheer him up or to shame or force him to resume activities of which he is not capable. These attempts evoke guilt, a feeling of inadequacy, and hostility in additional quanta which must be handled according to the psycho-dynamic pattern of the patient's illness and hence intensify the depression. Unless it is possible to obtain the rapid and whole-hearted co-operation of the relatives some type of hospitalization is essential to successful therapy. Occasional patients, early in a depressive illness, will become quite reckless in their social and business behavior in a last desperate attempt to assure themselves of their adequacy or to force greater satisfaction from the environment. Apparent acting-out in the sexual area to reassure the individual of potency or attractiveness may be prominent. An irrevocable, and often sacrificing, termination of business and financial interest may reflect both the patient's sense of hopelessness and his final, subtle expression of hostility. Certainly adequate measures must be taken to protect the patient from this type of destructive action toward himself and here too hospitalization may be indicated.

Many technics, programs and measures have been attempted for the treatment of depression, as indicated in Table 9. Favorable results have been claimed for all of these and almost all still have advocates.

An extensive survey of the literature on these various drugs and methods of treatment may be found in Bellak, but as this author comments, the reported efficacy of most of them could well be dependent on the increased amount of attention afforded the patient during their administration. However, there is no doubt of the value of a selected few in the accomplishment of the aims set forth in Table 8.

Sleep disturbance in the depressed patient is often most bitterly complained about. Sleep is restless and early awakening is most frequent, producing greater anxiety and hence less sleep. It is thus of great urgency to bring this symptom under control as quickly as possible. While hypnotic drugs may be necessary, their use should be limited both for avoidance of after-effects in debilitated patients and from consideration of increased tendency to dependency in these patients. They should be used if necessary after long neutral baths, massage, or other physiotherapeutic measures have

TABLE 9. METHODS UTILIZED IN THERAPY OF DEPRESSION

Measures for Physical Symptoms:	Principle Somatic Therapies:
Sedatives and hypnotics	Electroconvulsive therapy
Hydrotherapy (continuous baths)	Electronarcosis
Enemas and laxatives	Insulin coma therapy
Tube feeding	Insulin sub-coma therapy
	Metrazol convulsive therapy
Drugs and Hormones:	Continuous sleep treatment
Amphetamines	
Ephedrine	Other Somatic Technics:
Atropine	"Own blood" injections
Vitamins	Bilateral stellate ganglion blocks
(Niacin, nicotinic acid, et al.)	Refrigeration
Acetylcholine	Pyretotherapy (malaria)
Liver extracts	
Testosterone	Psychotherapeutic Measures:
Theelin and other estrogens	Occupational therapy
Eschatin	Psychodrama
Decholin	Group psychotherapy
Histamine	"Brief" psychotherapy
Ether (I.V.)	Psychoanalysis
Gynergen	
Hematoporphyrin	Psychosurgical Procedures:
Sulfapyradine	Lobotomy
Picrotoxin	Leucotomy
Reserpine	Thalamotomy
Chlorpromazine	Topectomy
Others	

failed. Chloral hydrate or Dormisone are often to be preferred over barbiturate drugs because of the more even and natural sleep they provide and the relative freedom from after-effects.

Improvement of nutritional status often commands immediate attention. The patient should be coaxed, tempted and, if necessary, spoon fed at frequent intervals with small morning, afternoon and bedtime nourishments. Simply setting food before the patient is more often than not quite insufficient, since retardation and feelings of unworthiness coupled with anorexia and various gastrointestinal complaints make it easier for the patient not to eat. In severe depressions tube feeding is often imperative. Nasal feeding is usually most satisfactory. Insofar as possible these feedings should be varied and contain a high carbohydrate, high protein diet, with milk, eggs, fruit juices, meat broths, strained vegetables and vitamin preparations. Such tube feeding may of course stir up the patient's antagonism and aversion and should not be continued any longer than necessary and frequent attempts at regular feeding should be made.

Constipation is another very up-setting problem to most depressed patients and considerable progress in establishing confidence and co-operation may be made by correction of this difficulty. In addition, the danger of impaction in the undernourished and dehydrated patient should not be overlooked. The physician should keep close watch on this matter and not rely on the vague reports of the patient. Treatment depends on the type of constipation, whether spastic or atonic. In the spastic colon nightly instillations of oil are often helpful and occasionally tincture of belladonna may bring relief. More frequently in depressions an atonic colon is encountered which responds to increased fluid intake, senna tea, mineral oil, cascara 0.4 to 0.6 Gm., or epsom salts 1 to 2 oz., depending on the severity of the condition. Enemas may be used if other measures are inadequate, but should be avoided if possible because of the psychological reaction in many patients.

In severe depressions attention must be paid to the general hygiene of the patient and the necessary assistance afforded for care of teeth, mouth, skin, hair, etc. Occasionally catheterization may become necessary.

When indicated, an appropriate form of somatic therapy should be started early after diagnosis is made and the need determined. Management of the physiologic problems discussed above is most frequently greatly facilitated by somatic therapy and improvement in this area is often the first evidence of effective therapy.

While a great variety of theories have been advanced to explain the mode of operation of the various somatic therapies, no one theory or combination of theories is adequate or well established at present. Table 10 summarizes several of the more important theories offered.[31]

More avid advocates of each of the various methods claim special advantages for their particular technic of somatic therapy. However, review of the results reported for insulin coma, metrazol convulsions and electroconvulsions used in the treatment of depressions indicates that if any therapeutic advantage exists it prob-

TABLE 10.   THEORIES OF SOMATIC THERAPIES

Neutralization or increased metabolism of hypothetical stimulant toxin (Sakel, Danziger).

Biologic antagonism of epileptic convulsions and schizophrenic illness (Meduna).

Organism brought to state near death, producing:

Maximal biologic defense reaction exerted through substance produced by brain (acroagonine of Cerletti). Pituitary and adrenal reaction to stress, with re-establishment of disturbed hormone balance (Sackler, Reiss and others).

Maximal mobilization of psychic defenses with break in autism and narcissism, and reappraisal of reality (Jelliffe and others).

Reduction in brain metabolism by anoxia or hypoglycemia produces:

Death of hypothetical diseased brain cells (Stief).

Compensatory increase in activity after treatment (Sereijski, Himwich and others).

Reflex stimulation of diencephalic neurovegetative centers and/or pituitary (Gellhorn and others).

Stimulation is primarily of the diencephalic neurovegetative centers (Ewald, Delay and Mallet, and others).

Therapies produce helpless dependence and increased attention thus facilitating transference and psychotherapy (Meier, Schatner and others).

Reaction to fear of treatment or to need for punishment (Rubenovitch, Mosse).

Temporary confusion and memory deficit allow impingement of problems at reduced rate allowing gradual integration.

More sensitive neural connections are temporarily interrupted:

More recent abnormal patterns "burned out" allowing return to former adjustment.

Recent (psychotic) defenses damaged, facilitating psychotherapy.

Connection of ideas (cortical) and affects (hypothalamic) interrupted reducing the "drive" of abnormal behavior.

ably favors electroconvulsive therapy. Metrazol convulsions produce no greater recovery rates and have the disadvantages of being more difficult to administer, less predictable and more liable to the production of complications. Insulin shows no consistent advantage and is much more expensive and difficult to produce. However, occasional patients with more marked schizoid, paranoid or anxiety features may prove refractory to convulsive treatments but respond to insulin coma alone or to combined coma and convulsive therapy.

In treatment of depression electroconvulsive treatment consistently proves of greater benefit than the nonconvulsive types of therapies such as continuous sleep treatment, electronarcosis, pyretotherapy, various drug and hormone therapies, or the more intensive types of psychotherapy used alone or in combinations excluding convulsive therapy. Increasing evidence is being presented that this statement may hold true even for the more psychogenic or neurotic depressions.[32, 33] However, careful evaluation of psychodynamic, social and economic factors in the individual patient must be the basis for deciding on the use of convulsive therapy in this type of depression. Various combinations of electroconvulsive treatments with other technics or drugs have been reported beneficial, but with the exception of the measures discussed, their usefulness in the treatment of depression is not yet established.

With convulsive therapy remission rates in depressive patients are variously reported between 80 and 100 per cent which roughly corresponds to the spontaneous remission rates for this same group. However, numerous studies indicate that the duration of the depressive episode and of hospitalization is reduced by from 70 to 80 per cent by the use of convulsive therapy. Suicide rates and readmission rates within one year of discharge appear to be reduced by approximately 50 per cent in the treated groups. At present there is no good evidence that convulsive treatment has any appreciable effect on the frequency of recurrences of depressive episodes, and aside from relapses during the first year after discharge there appears to be no significant effect on the duration of remission. Although, as it appears from these facts, convulsive treatment does not "cure" depressions and their underlying pathology, the savings both in human misery and in psychiatric resources are undeniable and inestimable.

Several different technics and types of equipment are utilized in administration of electroconvulsive therapy, the advantages or disadvantages of which are adequately discussed by Kalinowsky and Hoch.[31] The use of curare drugs to "soften the convulsion" and avoid complicating fractures and muscular injuries has long been a subject of some controversy since these drugs frequently resulted in apnea of considerable duration, a complication more dangerous than those avoided. Recently, however, short acting succinylcholine salts have been introduced for the production of muscle relaxation or paralysis during convulsive therapy. Since full recovery from the paralytic action usually occurs within five minutes, prolonged apnea is avoided. Usually this drug is administered in conjunction with an ultrashort-acting barbiturate which causes the patient to sleep (6 to 8 cc. of a 2.5 per cent solution thiopental sodium, i.v.), thus reducing the fear of the paralytic drug and of the treatment. After the patient is asleep the estimated dose of succinylcholine dichloride is then injected i.v. The dosage will vary with the muscle mass to be paralyzed, the degree of paralysis desired, the age of the patient, and probably other unknown factors, but will seldom be greater than 100 mg., averaging about 40 mg. Within a few seconds complete relaxation will be noted as indicated by free inflation of the lungs on compression of the rebreathing bag. The convulsive current is then applied and results in very mild clonic contractions of the feet, hands and face, occasionally spreading to other parts. Oxygen inflation of the lungs may be practiced during this stage. After cessation of the convulsion, the patient is turned on his side to allow elimination of any secretions, and artificial respiration is used until the return of the patient's own respirations. Only minimal complications have been reported with this technic and the usual skeletal and muscle complications of convulsive therapy are eliminated.[34]

With the barbiturate and succinylcholine technics, the co-operation of patients and relatives is much more easily maintained and much of the undesirable fear and postconvulsive discomfort is avoided. There is some indication that this method also reduces the postconvulsive confusion and amnesia which are quite troublesome in a few patients. Certainly these less "brutal" technics are easier on the sensibilities of the staff and the physician.

Contraindications to convulsive treatment have steadily been reduced in the past ten years, both by new technics such as that described above and by the increased realization of the advantages to be expected from convulsive treatment. If proper care is taken and special technics are used, it is now generally felt that increased intracranial pressure, aneurysm of the aorta, and possibly coronary disease are the only commonly encountered definite contraindications.

On the average, depressed patients will respond with good recovery to only four or five convulsive treatments but most physicians feel that an additional four to six treatments are of advantage for stabilization of the gains made. No definite pattern is widely followed in this matter.

The value of psychotherapy in the treatment of depressed patients, particularly those with so-called endogenous depressions, has frequently been seriously challenged. Certainly the rate of remission produced by psychotherapy without convulsive therapy in the more severe depressions has been most discouraging and in some cases appears less than the spontaneous remission rate. Some have suggested that even with convulsive treatment any attempt at other than the most superficial supportive and manipulative psychotherapy is a waste of time and may be harmful in severe endogenous depression. These impressions would be difficult to prove or disprove and it seems safe to say that most psychiatrists make some attempt to assist the depressed patient understand his illness in some psychodynamic terms, after the acute symptoms are brought under control. While it is the clinical impression of Kalinowsky that follow-up psychotherapy of depressed patients after convulsive therapy and discharge does not significantly effect prognosis with regard to recurrence when a past pattern of recurrence is demonstrable, this does not take into account either the quality of adjustment during remission or the suppression of a pattern of recurrence which might otherwise be evident.[35]

As indicated in Table 8 psychotherapy is adapted to the needs of the total management program and must be closely integrated with this program. During the severe depressive stages and before the physiologic symptoms are brought under some control, intensive psychotherapy is futile and may, if attempted, create greater resistance and aversion in the patient. The patient is in no position to offer the co-operation necessary for such therapy and may view attempts as another impossible demand and an imposition. A brief general outline of psychotherapy with depressed patients is found in Table 11. Utilization of such resources as occupational therapy, psychodrama, group sessions and social gatherings, and social work service can greatly facilitate the work of the psychotherapist.

Except for sedatives and hypnotics in the relief of sleep difficulties and laxatives in relief of constipation, few drugs are of proved value in the treatment of depression. The amphetamine group is

TABLE 11. PRINCIPLES OF PSYCHOTHERAPY IN DEPRESSION

Severe Phase:
  Frequent brief contacts (10 to 20 minutes, 2 to 4 times daily).
  Simple explanations of illness, patient attention to complaints followed by reassurance as to prognosis.
  Short superficial interpretive remarks widely spaced with plenty of time for assimilation and integration.
  Careful explanation of necessary procedures.
  Steady, tactful and gentle encouragement toward participiation in simple occupational therapy and other activities.
  Slow superficial investigation of disturbing environmental factors with early manipulative assistance where possible.
  No arguing or unnecessary forcing of opinions on patient.

Improved and Convalescent Phase:
  Progressive deepening of investigation with patient of disturbing life situations and clarification of typical patterns of reaction with possible alternatives.
  Assistance in ventilation of hostility.
  Recognition of dependency needs and assistance in acceptance of these needs through reassurance.
  Assistance in planning for return to home environment and discussion of problems involved including feelings about illness and hospitalization.

Follow-up Phase:
  Encouragement toward gradual resumption of normal responsibilities and activities.
  Continued exploration of reaction patterns and their meaning.
  Afford opportunity for continued ventilation of hostility.
  Exploration of possible precipitating or aggravating environmental factors.
  Gradual reduction of frequency of contact to "p.r.n." basis.
  Explanation of "danger signals."

widely used by some and may be of benefit in mild depressions treatable on an office basis, but many patients react to these drugs with feelings of increased tension, restlessness and irritability. Occasionally, when feelings of hopelessness and depression respond well to 5.0 mg. of an amphetamine drug on awakening and at lunch time, the addition of a small dose of a barbiturate may control the tension feelings without counteracting the desirable effect of the amphetamine drug. Long-term benefits from such drugs are not to be expected and continued use is not to be recommended.

Considerable hope was held for the use of reserpine and chlorpromazine in the treatment of depression. Unfortunately, the use of these drugs has proved of little benefit and not infrequently they result in a deepening of the depression. According to Hoch's findings only an occasional agitated depression of the involutional group, of all the depressive patients treated, showed some improvement with these drugs.[36]

Initial attacks of manic-depressive reactions are most likely to be depressive and to occur between the ages of 15 and 25 years.

TABLE 12.   PROGNOSTIC INDICATORS IN DEPRESSION

Favorable:	Unfavorable:
Single episode	Recurrent episode
Initial onset before age 30	Initial onset after age 40
Preponderance of environmental determinants	Strong hereditary history
	Hypochondriacal delusions
Mixed types	Schizoid pre-psychotic personality
Extroverted pre-psychotic personality	Persistent depersonalization
	Paranoid or suicidal trends
Predominantly "anal" character traits	Hallucinosis
	Predominantly "oral" character traits

Subsequent attacks show a distinct tendency toward increasing severity, duration and frequency. Prognostic signs in the single episode have been carefully studied and a number of tests and criteria presented by various workers (Table 12), but long-term prognosis presents considerably greater problems. It is apparent from preceding discussions that avoidance of recurrent attacks has not been significantly effected by present therapies, insofar as can be ascertained from existing statistics. Certainly more study, carefully controlled, directed toward evaluation of measures for the prevention of recurrences is desperately needed. At present, it can only be hoped that improvement in psychotherapeutic methods both during and after hospitalization will make possible optimal adjustment during remissions and increase the likelihood that the patient may be able to avoid precipitating factors. Educative measures in psychotherapy may also contribute by alerting the patient to danger signs, thus enabling earlier therapy. Continuous though irregular contacts with the patient during long-term follow-up will also make for earlier therapy and almost certainly reduce the severity of any recurrence. Electroconvulsive therapy used prophylactically in office practice appears to be of definite benefit in many cases. Educative efforts with relatives and associates of patients, when tactfully carried through, may considerably improve the long-term prognosis through the improvement of environmental satisfactions to the patient.

SUMMARY

1. The history of concepts concerning depressive illnesses, their cause and treatment, is reviewed.

2. Various classifications of depressive illness and their differentiation are presented. It is suggested that mental illness is related on two independent continua: one from pure psychogenicity to pure organicity, and the second in terms of degree of integration.

3. The etiology of manic-depressive depression is not definitely established and at present the best statement which can be made is that the illness is a reaction to psychobiologic stress in an individual predisposed by varying combinations of constitutional and psychodynamic factors.

4. Symptoms of depression are presented.

5. Psychodynamic configurations are presented.

6. Methods of therapy and various theories of their mode of action are presented. It can be stated that therapy at present is entirely empirical. Electroconvulsive therapy is best established as beneficial, but has no established effect on the duration of remissions unless used in a prophylactic manner during remissions.

7. General prinicples of management, of psychotherapy and of follow-up are discussed.

BIBLIOGRAPHY

1. Burton, Robert: The Anatomy of Melancholy, New York, Tudor, 1938.
2. Zilboorg, G., and Henry G.: A History of Medical Psychology, New York, Norton, 1941.
3. Jelliffe, S. E.: in Manic-Depressive Psychosis, Vol. XI Series of

Research Publications, A. Research Nerv. & Ment. Dis. Proc., Baltimore, Williams & Wilkins, 1931.

4. Kraepelin, E.: Manic-Depressive Insanity and Paranoia, Trans. by R. Mary Barclay and Ed. by George M. Robertson, Edinburgh, Livingstone, 1921.

5. Abraham, Karl: Notes on the Psycho-Analytical Investigation and Treatment of Manic-Depressive Insanity and Allied Conditions (1911). Selected Papers on Psycho-Analysis, London, Hogarth Press, 1948.

6. Freud, Sigmund: Mourning and Melancholia (1917). Collected Papers, London, Hogarth Press, 1946.

7. Rado, Sandor: The problem of melancholia, Internat. J. Psychoan. 9:420, 1928.

8. ————: Hedonic Control, Action-Self, and the Depressive Spell. In Depression, Ed. Hoch and Zubin, New York, Grune & Stratton, 1954.

9. Kretschmer, E.: Heredity and constitution in aetiology of psychic disorders, Brit. Med. J. 2:403, 1937.

10. Sheldon, W. H., Stevens, S. S., and Tucker, W. B.: The Varieties of Human Physique, New York, Harper, 1940.

11. Lasker, G. W.: The effects of partial starvation on somatotype. An analysis of material from the Minnesota starvation experiment, Am. J. Phys. Anthropol. 5:323, 1947.

12. White, William A.: Outlines of Psychiatry, ed. 10, Washington, Nervous & Mental Disease Publishing Co., 1924.

13. Bellak, L.: Manic-Depressive Psychosis and Allied Conditions, New York, Grune & Stratton, 1952.

14. Fenichel, Otto: The Psychoanalytic Theory of Neurosis, New York, Norton, 1945.

15. Henderson, David, and Gillespie, R. D.: A Text-Book of Psychiatry, ed. 7, London, Oxford, 1950.

16. Strecker, E. A., Ebaugh, F. G., and Ewalt, J. R.: Practical Clinical Psychiatry, ed. 7, Philadelphia, Blakiston, 1951.

17. Noyes, Arthur P.: Modern Clinical Psychiatry, ed. 4, Philadelphia, Saunders, 1953.

18. Slater, E. T. O.: The inheritance of manic-depressive insanity, Proc. Roy. Soc. Med. 29:981, 1936.

19. Kallmann, Franz J.: Genetic Principles in Manic-Depressive Psychosis. In Depression, Ed. Hoch and Zubin, New York, Grune & Stratton, 1954.

20. Campbell, J. D.: Manic-Depressive Disease, Philadelphia, Lippincott, 1953.

21. Lewis, Nolan D. C., and Piotrowski, Zygmunt A.: Clinical Diagnosis of Manic-Depressive Psychosis. In Depression, Ed. Hoch and Zubin, New York, Grune & Stratton, 1954.

22. McFarland, R. A., and Goldstein, H.: The biochemistry of manic-depressive psychosis, Am. J. Psychiat. **96**:21, 1939.
23. Reiss, Max: Investigations of Hormone Equilibria During Depression. *In* Depression, Ed. Hoch and Zubin, New York, Grune & Stratton, 1954.
24. Sackler, Arthur M., Sackler, Raymond R., Marti-Ibanez, Feliz, and Sackler, Mortimer D.: Contemporary physiodynamic trends in psychiatry, J. Clin. Exper. Psychopath. & Quart. Rev. Psy. & Neuro. **15**:382, 1954.
25. Klopfer, B., and Kelley, D. McG.: The Rorschach Technique, New York, World, 1942.
26. Travis, J. H.: Precipitating factors in manic-depressive psychoses, Psychiat. Quart. **7**:411, 1933.
27. Brew, M. F.: Precipitating factors in manic-depressive psychosis, Psychiat. Quart. **7**:401, 1933.
28. Oltman, J. E., and Friedman, S.: The role of operative procedure in the etiology of psychosis, Psychiat. Quart. **17**:405, 1943.
29. Diethelm, Oskar: Treatment in Psychiatry, ed. 2, Springfield, Thomas, 1950.
30. Wall, J. H.: The psychiatric problem of suicide, Am. J. Psychiat. **101**:404, 1944.
31. Kalinowsky, L. B., and Hoch, Paul H.: Shock Treatments, Psychosurgery and Other Somatic Treatments in Psychiatry, New York, Grune & Stratton, 1952.
32. Myerson, A.: Prolonged cases of grief reaction treated by electric shock, New England J. Med. **230**:253, 1944.
33. Davidoff, Eugene, and Zack, Russ, Jr.: The Treatment of Various Types of Depression in a General Hospital. *In* Depression, Ed. Hoch and Zubin, New York, Grune & Stratton, 1954.
34. Steven, R. J. M., Tovell, R. M., Johnson, J. C., and Delegado, Enrique: Anesthesia for electroconvulsive therapy, Anesthesiol. **15**:623, 1954.
35. Kalinowsky, L. B.: Some Problems in Electric Convulsive Therapy of Depressions. *In* Depressions, Ed. Hoch and Zubin, New York, Grune & Stratton, 1954.
36. Hoch, Paul H.: The Effect of Chlorpromazine on Moderate and Mild Mental and Emotional Disturbances. *In* Chlorpromazine and Mental Health, Philadelphia, Lea & Febiger, 1955.

THE MANAGEMENT OF EMOTIONAL
REACTIONS IN THE MALE
INVOLUTIONAL PERIOD

Otto Billig, M.D.

When I first became interested in the subject of the emotional problems of the middle-aged man I found very little about it in the professional literature. However, a few publications appeared during the last two or three years. In considering the problem of middle age or of the climacteric period we are apt to associate it with the woman rather than with the man. I wonder if the sex and the age of the majority of professional writers may have something to do with such one-sidedness. We are always more hesitant to look at ourselves in the mirror in the fear of discovering our own wrinkles; writers on psychiatric subjects do not seem an exception to this.

The problem of middle age has customarily been approached from an endocrine point of view; there has been considerable thought given to the dysfunction of the various endocrine glands. A recent editorial in the *Journal of the American Medical Association*,[9] "Is there a true male climacteric?" has thrown some important light on the subject. Some of the quoted authors are more inclined to accept an endocrine explanation of the problem but the editorial writer stresses the lack of conclusive evidence for such an assumption. He emphasizes that the true male climacteric is a rare condition and only infrequently demonstrated by laboratory tests or relieved by substitution therapy. The supposedly characteristic symptoms for the male or female climacteric are not at all specific. The patients are described as being anxious, somewhat depressed, irritable and having feelings of inadequacy. But such subjective symptoms are found in all types of emotional disturbances. The J.A.M.A. editorial concludes by warning against the "promiscuous use of male hormone," considering it "unwarranted and . . . harmful."

Possibly the definition of the term "climacterium" may give some additional leads to its meaning and significance. The literal translation of climacterium means "top round of a ladder," the climax. According to ancient Chinese writers, there are seven periods of life where the top round of the ladder is reached, necessitating a readjustment to life situations. Such times are, for instance, not only adolescence, marriage, but also middle age. In all of those periods a deep-going emotional readjustment becomes necessary. It is this adaptation to new life situations that may be of significance in our problem. Since the changes in the physical and chemical conditions of the body do not seem to lead to any conclusive evidence, we should possibly examine the changes in the social and cultural structure of the individual's environment.

The social, scientific, political and philosophical structure of our society has undergone far-reaching changes during the last 150 years. Traditional social goals have been abandoned. The Dutch historian, J. Huizinga,[7] describes the medieval society as having clearly marked objectives accepted by all its people without dispute. It resulted in renunciation of the individual's interests and in salvation through his suffering. A feeling of security was attained through group identification. The society of those days was authoritarian and patriarchal. Science, if we can apply the term, was not allowed to question established beliefs. Strength was given through a rigid dogma and arbitrarily stated assumptions. Society reacted quickly and strongly against scientific discoveries outside of the narrowly outlined dogma. It was intuitively recognized that such developments would shake the medieval social structure. Both the church and secular power protected the authority of the existing social structure. During the Inquisition, they collaborated in suppressing anything that might question their authority. The discovery of the earth not being the center of the universe resulted in near panic. If the earth was no longer the center of the universe around which all the other stars rotated, so the king soon may not be considered as the center of his empire. It was attempted to suppress such views as heresy. But the concepts of the medieval man and his philosophies had to change through the consistent force of the new discoveries. During the subsequent years an increasing importance was placed on the significance of the individual having far-reaching social and political implications. The old master had lost his power. New scientific systems revealed revolutionary vistas for everyone. The newly found order and structure of the world made the individual's frontiers almost limitless. The subsequent development of communication brought us closer to our neighbors. New opportunities stimulated aspirations and brought achievements within the reach of many. But soon such possibilities conflicted with others. The individual began to collide with his fellow man. His close relationship to his neighbors and his knowing of this relationship produced anxiety about their nature and intentions. Competition became emphasized. Since the goals came within the reach of many, each individual became aware of others being in the race. Kardiner[10] considers the nineteenth century as a period of opportunities and discoveries, but the increasing competition of the twentieth century makes those opportunities shrink again. What effect did this new development have on the individual's outlook and adjustment? It shifted the emphasis onto himself; he became all important; he felt that he could reach and achieve unlimited goals. The goals were close. His life was made easier through the development of science and the machines but he began to recognize that those machines made him dispensable. What he had accomplished in many days and weeks before, could be easily done in a few hours now by pushing a button on one of his new creations. He became fearful of the things he had built. On the one hand, he was able to find satisfactions not known before, on the other, he became increasingly aware of others reaching for the same satisfactions and interfering with his achievements. The individual became more powerful and in some ways more significant but also more fearful of losing his newly found significance and dignity as man.

The family resisted the outside changes longest. But finally, the change in the role of the individual, his anxiety and his fear of losing his dignity, became reflected in the family. Not only that the king had lost his hold on authority, but also the master in his own home was beginning to lose his power. The father no longer was able to maintain the unquestioned significance that he had up to 50 or 100 years ago. This is shown in today's chronicles of the comic strip and the TV program. "Life with Father" indicates adequately the gradual change that came with the late nineteenth century; and Dagwood is a helpless, insignificant man who is always outsmarted by his wife. Are those caricatures entirely without basis or are they indicative of changes in the family structure? They may ridicule some of the weaknesses of our society but is there some foundation to them?

Families particularly susceptible to the competitions of our society tend to defend themselves with the stereotypes of mass culture.[10] Such groups exercise a sensitive role in the community usually belonging to a social "fringe" or minority group. Their members are sensitive to the achievement level of the community and eager to conform. The father may work hard to maintain his everyday responsibilities, spending little time at home. He needs to compete continuously in order to convince himself of his success. He never actually masters his fears of being replaced. His insecurities lead to painful feelings of inadequacies or to an attempt to compensate in the form of overconfidence. Having in his own mind failed to meet the demands of his job he does not consider himself an adequate provider for his family. If he does not receive sufficient emotional support at home he soon becomes ineffective in the opinion of himself. Others in the family recognize his overt anxieties or false attempts to assert his masculine "superiority."

The actual extent of the intrafamily frictions can be modified by the part of the mother. A sound and mature personality will add stability to the family even if the father functions on an inadequate level. But if the mother is unable to accept her own role increased tensions will result. The emotionally immature woman unconsciously envies the man. She undermines his position by criticisms and demands that he cannot meet. She expresses increasing dissatisfaction with her marriage, making unfavorable comparisons between her own life and that of her neighbors or other members of the family; often, she converts unconsciously her emotional disappointments into physical complaints. Dissatisfied with her marriage she tries to find fulfillment of her phantasies in her children. The children become aware of having to live up to the parents' high expectations. They have to please if they want to

feel loved; mother's love is conditioned on success in the class-
room, on the football team, in the social group. It is not only
important to acquire knowledge in their schoolwork, but possibly
more important to outrank others in the class standing. The young
boy has not only to be accepted in a fraternity but has to choose
his friends properly so that it will be the best fraternity. Soon, the
youngster develops insecurities about his achievements and doubts
if he would be able to continue to compete successfully. He feels
under constant pressure to "jockey" for position. Competition becomes the motivating force both outside the family and within.
Thus, rivalry among the siblings develops.

The following case history may illustrate such a family relationship.

A 43-year-old successful university professor develops hypertension;
moderate depression and anxiety follow the administration of one of
the new antihypertensive medications. The patient's sleep becomes disturbed, feelings of inadequacy and of not being able to fulfill the job
requirements appear. Having reached a recognized academic position,
he assumes that he fooled his co-workers and is actually not as capable
as others consider him to be.

Past history reveals that the father had a minor position in a bank.
Although a hard worker, he was never successful and basically ineffective. He did not feel secure in his work, always fearful of being fired or
replaced by a younger worker. The mother was continuously dissatisfied
and felt that the family could not afford as many little luxuries as her
sisters. She expressed openly keen disappointment with her marriage,
with having been unfortunate to marry a man who had not achieved
more.

The patient is the older of two boys, the younger sibling being the
patient's junior by two years. The patient had the impression that the
mother was partial to the younger brother and held him up as a model
for the patient to imitate. The patient recalled the painful insecurities
about his scholastic achievements and he never felt sure of pleasing
his teachers, developing disturbing anxiety especially toward his women
teachers.

The mother undermined the father's position by pointing out his
inability to earn an adequate living for the family. When the patient
needed money for school activities, the mother never failed to mention
that she was unable to give him the money because of the father's
inadequate income. The father's activities made it difficult for him to
spend much time with the boy. He became dependent on the mother's
approval; he recognized early in life that he had to live up to her
expectations if he wanted her acceptance. But the mother was never

entirely satisfied with the patient, always reminding him of his brother's more outgoing and more affectionate manner.

The patient started working early in life, contributing to the family's support. He had only a little time to play with youngsters of his own age; he felt timid with girls, appearing shy and withdrawn. He married a supportive and understanding woman fairly early in life. His wife assumed management of the family affairs and finances. The patient willingly turned those matters over to her; however, criticizing her for not being able to take care of things adequately and spending too much money. In spite of promotions in his job he remained uncertain if he would be able to continue in his work or if he would not be asked for his resignation. His apparent outstanding work record and continued recognition from his superiors were not reassuring to him.

Summary. This patient was brought up by a controlling, domineering mother. She blocked the patient's need to establish a satisfactory relationship with his father by undermining his authority. The young boy was not able to identify with an adequate male figure. This encouraged his dependency on his mother and similar women figures. The mother's personality made him fearful of powerful women adding to his difficulties in assuming a secure masculine role. His unsuccessful attempts to compete with his brother—a competition that was unconsciously encouraged by the mother—increased his feelings of inadequacies and of being replaced by more successful men. These mechanisms made him more vulnerable to feeling attacked at middle age—at a time when the cultural pattern intensifies such conflicts.

The father's ineffective role is not caused only by the obvious insecurities and lack of assertiveness. His inability to prepare the son to meet the demands of society may be shown by the next case.

The patient is a 40-year-old professional worker who comes to the office since he feels unable to "adjust himself to life." He complains of losing his temper easily and of becoming increasingly aware of a strong resentment against his wife and his two sons. He has felt depressed over fairly long periods of times and has been insecure in his work.

His father is in his sixties, foreign born, very successful in his business as a wholesale grocery man. He was always demanding, highly critical and had violent temper outbursts. He was a hard worker, ambitious and greatly concerned with proving himself through his financial success. This was particularly important to him since he belonged to a minority group. He spent a great deal of time in his store. Starting on a small basis, he was able to build a large undertaking.

The patient's mother is described as a quiet woman, always anxious to have peace at home. But the patient resented her permitting herself to be controlled by the patriarchal father. The patient never felt that the mother was able to give him adequate support against the outbursts of his father. He considered his childhood and particularly his adolescence as very unhappy. He was not able to study in school, failed and finally dropped out of school for three years. He worked in his father's grocery store during that period. He re-entered high school upon the advice of a kind, fatherly minister. The father originally opposed the patient's returning to school but finally consented. While still in high school, the patient met his later wife. The girl had already finished college, was very popular with other young people and had several chances of marrying promising young men. The patient dated his wife for several years, the wife being the aggressor. They finally married before the patient's graduation. The father opposed the marriage. The wife worked to contribute to the young couple's support. After five years she became pregnant. The first pregnancy was planned. The patient commented: "It gave me a masculine feeling." During the wife's pregnancy he had two extramarital affairs. The second pregnancy occurred two months after the first child was born. The patient was very much disturbed over this second pregnancy and very much irritated at his wife for not having prevented it. Again, he entered extramarital affairs, this time, with the feeling that he was justified in doing so by his wife's making life difficult for him.

After the last delivery, the couple got along fairly well until about two years ago. The patient had become increasingly depressed over his concern that his "life would be almost completely over" when he reached 40 years of age. The patient referred to his sex life, saying that he had been always preoccupied with sex and that he had been fearful of a decreasing sexual capacity. During these last two years there had been increasing quarreling at home, primarily over money matters. The wife had stopped working when she became pregnant for the first time. The patient felt that she should have continued to contribute to the support of the family. Another source for disagreements was the increasing disciplinary problems involving their two sons. His relationship with his older (12 years old) son had been particularly poor. The patient, never satisfied with him, criticized and nagged continuously. The son increased the patient's conflicts by asking if he, the patient, hated him. The patient realized that his son felt about him as he had felt about his own father.

Following the domestic encounters, the patient had phantasies of going on trips from which he would not return home. He became increasingly concerned about financial matters, blaming himself for not being able to be more successful in finding adequate security for himself and his family. He blamed it on not choosing the right profession since there was "no money in my profession." He began to realize that he was motivated in his choice of his particular profession by his apparent rebellion against the father's business. He wanted to remove himself as far as possible from the father's type of business. However, in more recent years he had phantasies of returning to his home town as a successful man.

Soon after entering therapy the patient reported one of his first dreams. The patient and his wife were in an apartment. They "were both standing around. I had the impression that we were just married. A friend came in and snatched some abstract decorations that were on all the pieces of furniture. Those decorations were made of cigars—no, of pipe cleaners. They were long, bent objects. After he snatched those decorations, he laughed hilariously and walked out with them." The patient associated a recent discussion he had with his wife. The wife started talking about doing some substitute teaching. She based this desire on "we have to recognize the actual reality of our situation. Your job doesn't pay enough and so I had better start contributing something." The patient became very upset over the wife's remarks. "She wanted to point out my inefficiencies and my inability to earn enough money. It only makes me more hostile." The patient made those remarks after having mentioned that he had talked previously with his wife about taking a job.

Summary. This patient had considerable difficulty in his relationship to his father whom he always thought of as very controlling and wanting to have "his way at all cost." The patient felt that his father considered him to be "a weakling and an inadequate person." Strong hostile feelings and death wishes against the father moved close to the surface of his emotional adjustment. He was unable to identify himself with the rejecting father resulting in difficulties in assuming a masculine role. His mother appeared to him as unable to defend him against the father. In spite of some strong attachment to the mother, he felt basically rejected by her. His choice of a marital partner was greatly influenced by his conflictual relationship to the mother. He married a supportive woman of whom he could expect that she would help by working if this should become necessary. The patient became emotionally disturbed by his wife's pregnancies. It reactivated his conflicts about the father's role. He attempted to deny his being married by having extramarital relationships. When he approached middle age he developed increased anxieties and depressive symptoms. He must have unconsciously recalled his hostile feelings toward his father and he attempted to protect himself by wanting to continue in the father's footsteps. The father's controlling and all-powerful role within the family appeared to give protection against any underlying insecurities. But through his identification with his father he became increasingly aware of his own difficulties with his sons, stating frankly that "my son has the same relation with me that I had with my father. I become just as unreasonably angry with him as my father did with me." When he unconsciously felt his hostile feelings toward his father, he feared the same response in his older son toward him. This caused him to become anxious and depressed.

The father in the last case was ineffective in his relationship to his son. The reason was entirely different from the first one. The father attempted to defend himself against his own insecurities by hard work and a strict, patriarchal attitude. He demanded blind obedience from his sons and felt very easily threatened in his authority. He insisted on the unquestioned position as the head of the family and could never accept being in the wrong. He had to maintain his own masculine position by proving himself in competition with others. His need was met by being financially successful. He worked hard and accumulated money by his frugal means. Money became a power and symbol through which he hoped to buy love, affection and respect.

The father-son relationship has found its symbolic expression in the Oedipus conflict. This complex has been traced to the beginning of classical literature. It expresses a common conflict having universal application. Psychiatrists have recognized the significance of this complex as a basis for gaining an understanding of one's adjustment during childhood, adolescence and early adulthood. In an earlier publication,[3] we described a young man who developed a marked emotional disturbance at the time of his wife's second pregnancy. The first pregnancy had resulted in a spontaneous abortion. The young man was apparently emotionally unprepared for his wife's second pregnancy and wanted her to have an induced abortion. As the time of delivery approached the patient became increasingly disturbed, apparently about his own hostile impulses against the yet unborn child. We showed in this case that this patient himself had a good many unpleasant experiences with his father. Therefore, he had not been able to identify himself with a mature, accepting father role. In Sophocles' original play of Oedipus Rex young king Laius becomes frightened by the oracle's prediction of suffering his death through his son's hand when "the silver [is] just lightly strewn among his hair"—less poetically expressed, at middle age. In an attempt to circumvent his fate Laius decides to have his son killed. We consider this very reaction essential in creating anxiety at the time of expecting fatherhood of those who have not been able to establish a secure masculine role. Apparently they remember unconsciously the inadequate emotional relationship that existed between them and their own fathers. A recent study[5] of 55 "expectant fathers" indicated that about 60 per cent of them had marked difficulties at the time of the wife's pregnancies. It was concluded that those men had conflicts about their identification with their fathers. This hostility against the father is reactivated when a child is born anticipating an identical reaction from their newborn child. That time comes when their son reaches adulthood or the father enters middle age. If the original Oedipus conflict remains unresolved, we expect emotional difficulties (1) at the time of the birth of a child and (2) in middle age when the real or symbolic son reaches maturity and becomes sufficiently powerful to displace the father. The threats of this period are beginning to be recognized as sufficiently important in our competitive society to require protection of the middle-aged man from the young competitor: i.e., it was attempted to extend the Fair Employment Practice Law in New York State to exclude discrimination because of age. Bergler[2] describes a number of competitively successful men who develop emotional difficulties during middle age. Those men sought to handle their conflicts by an attempt to prove their masculinity in extramarital relationships. Bergler relates this to the mother's conditioned love during childhood resulting in the child feeling rejected. The son attempts to revenge those feelings of rejection through extramarital relations at the time of middle age. Meerloo[11] interprets problems of middle age as aggressive feelings turned against one's self. This results in self-destructive tendencies in the form of misuse of alcohol or drugs, hypochondriacal concern and self-pity. We had an occasion to study 150 men of a low competitive society. They had been admitted to the Vanderbilt University Hospital for persistent incapacitating illnesses of various etiology. One hundred patients were between the ages of 35 and 55 years; about 55 per cent of these had clear-cut emotional illnesses, mostly anxiety or conversion reactions with depressive features. An additional third had psychosomatic illnesses in which an emotional factor played a major part, and only 15 per cent had definite organic illnesses or complaints. The case histories were almost identical. The patients had been able to make a fairly good adjustment until they met with a minor illness or injury, when they became incapacitated. Apparently the minor interferences with the patient's health proved to be a great threat in the adjustment of those individuals. Each of these patients came from a very culturally restricted, narrow environment; the land was barren, the patients and their families seldom went to town and had little emotional satisfaction outside their work. They were raised in a strict church. The family relationships mirrored the cultural limitations. The typical father of this group was a very strict, austere person. The mother felt tied down by a large family; she had a good many complaints as to her health and found little time for the children. Affection was seldom expressed. The patients had early emotional difficulties in the form of neuropathic traits or "nervous habits." School attendance was irregular and terminated at an early age. The low income and the large family necessitated the children's starting to work. During adolescence, they tried to rebel against authority resulting in minor difficulties with the law. They married early; adjustment problems in marriage were common. The young husbands paid little attention to their wives and preferred "to run around with the boys." Several children were born in quick succession. The young fathers "settled down" in their late 20's and early 30's. They identified with their own fathers and became as strict as their fathers were with them. Soon they began to be health conscious, becoming increasingly preoccupied with their physical condition.

The emotional conflicts between father and son do not necessarily result in definite clinical symptoms but they can influence the attitudes and cultural patterns of a group. Reik[12] has related the ritual of the couvade to this kind of conflict. Among many primitive tribes the father is supposed to remain completely inactive at the time of his wife's delivery. This inactivity is to protect the unborn child from hostile impulses of the father. When the child became sick, it was considered due to the father's violation of the ritual inactivity. The father had to perform certain sacrifices in order to undo the harm done by his having been active.

South American tribes believe that the child is the reincarnation of the grandfather.[12] The grandfather is called the little father. In tribal ceremonies, the Indian man seeks protection from the fear that the grandfather came to life in the grandchild. And he fears that the hostility against his own father is avenged by his child.

The cruelties of the initiation ceremonies among primitives reveal the attempt of the older man to make the acceptance of the younger man as difficult as possible. The older men attempt to keep the "unfitted" youngster out of their group and many of the ceremonies are only ill-disguised cruelties against the novice. During the ritual he goes through the process of symbolic rebirth. The novice, when he becomes a fully accepted adult member of his group, is not permitted to mention the names of his family.[6] This protective forgetfulness prevents him from contacts with his father and mother. The hazing by medieval guilds or modern fraternities is reminiscent of such conflicts among Western civilizations.

The man who has emotional difficulties and conflicts during middle age seems to be a person who has not been able to resolve his conflict with his own father. The father appears ineffective either because of obvious, manifested insecurities, a lack of assertiveness or through overassertion and overemphasis of his own masculinity and patriarchal role. They may seek compensation for their insecurities in overemphasizing the importance of their masculine status in outdoor activities. Those are the men who prove themselves by constantly pointing to their capacity for physical endurance. Their exaggerated devotion and worship of sports almost convinces them that they can attain perpetual youth from such activities.

When married such men desire boys for their children. They consider having daughters as a reflection on their masculinity. If they should have girls, they become very protective of them and exhibit particular concern upon the girls entering adolescence. Such fathers insist on their patriarchal prerogative in protecting their daughters from the potential danger of a date with boys.

Their relationship to their sons is characterized by their own fear of life. They seldom fail to mention that "life is not a bed of roses" and set out to prepare their sons vigorously for it. In doing so the father rationalizes his own inability to accept his son readily. Very often the father shows contempt for the son's activities and demands his rights. "The American father brought up in the tradition of the pioneers, hardened in the period of rugged individualism, absorbed in the creation of material wealth, often looks down contemptuously upon his son's interest in history, literature or even theoretical physics. He considers such inclinations as a sign of decline, particularly if they do not produce adequate 'material rewards.' "[1] On the other hand, the father who prides himself on intellectual achievements may not be able to accept his son's lack of interest in such accomplishments and chides the son for his interest in superficial values rather than in "the more serious" aspects of life. The specific attitudes of the fathers vary but the basic mechanisms of not accepting the son and his interest remain the same.

In other cases, the father may attempt to compensate for his underlying unacceptance of his son. Then, he becomes overprotective and oversolicitous. At the same time, he is unable to tolerate the emancipation of his children. We described a case in which the father became emotionally disturbed at the time of the marriage of his daughters. When the young couple wanted to move away, the father attempted to keep them through all possible promises. He finally became psychotically disturbed when all attempts failed.

Other defenses against the anxiety of the middle-aged man may result in attempting to glamorize youth patterns and rising success. In such cases the older man becomes the sponsor of youth movements and attempts by all possible means to pacify the potential threat of the younger man by making him dependent on him.

The treatment management of the middle-aged man has to focus on the cause of his difficulties. As already pointed out, there is very little evidence to support an endocrine basis for the emotional difficulties of the middle-aged man. A deficiency of male hormone has not been established and there seems to be considerable doubt as to such an assumption.[4, 13, 14] If we accept the emotional factors as being of outstanding importance our treatment has to center in helping the patient in an emotional readjustment. Meerloo wrote that completely resolving the underlying complex does not seem to be indicated in the middle-aged man. He feels that the conflicts can be best handled by permitting the patient to establish an adequate relationship with the therapist. In doing so the fear of parental authority which originally existed may be resolved. It has been our own experience that the middle-aged man requiring psychiatric help shows greater than usual dependency needs. He tests the therapeutic relationship by asking for continued advice. By doing so, he needs to reassure himself that the therapist will not re-activate the role of the authoritative parent. At the same time, the patient will feel easily rejected if he does not receive the superficially desired reassurance. Psychotherapy progresses often considerably slower than in other cases of similar intellectual ability and cultural background.

Another factor of importance seems to be in helping the patient to achieve a secure role in the family. The emphasis on team relations seems to be essential. Each member of the family team needs to have a defined and circumscribed role, not threatening the other members of the team. Therefore, it is important to work with other members of the family. Social casework with the patient's wife may be of great help, especially if we realize that the original choice of a marital partner was very much determined by the patient's neurotic needs. The wife may have had difficulties in her own feminine role and even after the husband's difficulties are resolved, the wife would continue with her neurotic needs if she does not receive help. In some cases psychotherapy of the patient's wife will be essential.

Organic treatments, such as electric shock treatments, are of questionable success in the middle-aged man. We have attempted to treat a few cases of depression of middle age with electroshock therapy. Only temporary improvement was produced and those patients relapsed soon after the treatments were discontinued. In other cases treated with convulsive therapy confusional states resulted complicating the course of recovery. During such confusional states, the patients appeared disoriented, were untidy and had inadequate contact with their surroundings. The memory defect accompanying electroconvulsive therapy was more marked than usual. There was severe excitement present. Those conditions cleared spontaneously after electric shock treatments were discontinued.

In concluding I want to re-emphasize that the goals of psychotherapy are necessarily limited in treating the middle-aged man. The development of more mature self-evaluation through insight into his parental relationships, a better understanding of his marital relationships and the relationship to his own children seem to be the essential goal.

BIBLIOGRAPHY

1. Alexander, Franz: Discussion of: "Family problems and psychological disturbances." International Congress on Mental Health, London, 1948.
2. Bergler, Edmund: The Revolt of the Middle-Aged Man. New York, Wyn, 1954.
3. Billig, O., and Adams, R. W.: Emotional problems of the middle-aged man, Psychiat. Quart. 28:442, 1954.
4. Lansing, Albert (ed.): Cowdry's Problems of Aging, Baltimore, Williams & Wilkins, 1952.
5. Curtis, J. L.: A psychiatric study of 55 expectant fathers, U. S. Armed Forces M. J. 6:937, 1955.
6. Freud, S.: Totem and Taboo. Basic Writings of Sigmund Freud, New York, Modern Library, 1938.
7. Huizinga, J.: The Waning of the Middle Ages, Garden City, Doubleday, 1954.
8. Jones, E.: The Phantasy of the Reversal of Generations. Papers on Psychoanalysis, ed. 5, Baltimore, Williams & Wilkins, 1949.
9. Editorial: Is there a true male climacteric? J.A.M.A. 155:1427, 1945.
10. Kardiner, A.: Sex and Morality, Indianapolis, Bobbs-Merrill, 1954.
11. Meerloo, J. A. M.: Transference and resistance in geriatric psychotherapy, Psychoanalyt. Rev. 42:72, 1955.
12. Reik, Theodor: The Ritual: Psychoanalytic Studies, New York, Farrar, Straus, 1946.
13. Werner, August A.: The male climacteric, J.A.M.A. 127:705, 1945.
14. ———: The male climacteric, J.A.M.A. 132:188, 1946.

THE MANAGEMENT OF THE
MULTIPLE COMPLAINER

George C. Ham, M.D.

It is often quite useful when approaching the discussion of any subject, once the general heading has been chosen, to turn to definitions as found in standard dictionaries to obtain some clarification of the meaning of the words involved. If one turns in *Webster's New Collegiate Dictionary* to the word *complain* we find that it is derived from the French *com* plus the Latin *plangere* meaning *to strike, beat the breast in grief, or lament*. The two definitions that are given of its use in English are, first, *to give utterance to grief, pain, and discontent, etc.*, and second, *to make formal accusation or charge*. If we keep these meanings and the derivation in mind, it will be interesting to see how our present understanding of the dynamics of personality operation are so well expressed in meanings derived before such dynamic understanding of human behavior had been formulated. If one then turns to the definition of *manage*, we find that there are two derivations, one from the Latin and French words meaning *to manage*, and one from the Latin and French words meaning *hand*. It is also pointed out that in English the word has been influenced by the French *ménage* meaning housekeeping. One of the definitions that follows is *to control and direct; to conduct; to guide; to administer*. Another definition is *to render and keep (one) submissive; to wield with address*. A further definition is *to treat with care; to husband;* and another, *to bring about by contriving; to contrive*. An interesting colloquial synonym is the meaning: *to achieve one's purpose*.

It is interesting to note that all of these various definitions are applicable to the problem under discussion. It makes a great deal of difference, however, whether one is looking at this state of affairs from the position of the patient, the family, society or the doctor. Depending on the position in which one finds oneself in relation to the "complainer," one may want *to control,* or *to render (one) submissive,* or *to treat with care,* or *to contrive,* or *to achieve one's purpose* which may or may not be to the patient's interest. Returning for a moment to the patient, the patient may be wanting *to give utterance to some grief, or pain, or discontent,* or *may wish to make a formal accusation or charge.* Put in its most simple terms then, the "management" of the multiple complainer is the problem of interaction between an individual and one or more other individuals in various types of social interaction. It is an attempt of the "complainer" to communicate with those around him for purposes of gratification of need, and an attempt of the "managers" to understand and respond to these needs. Understanding has to precede response if the needs of the complainer are to be met. Ruesch and Bateson state that "Communication (includes) all those processes by which people influence one another. All actions and events have communicative aspects, as soon as they are perceived by a human being." Thus in dealing with a subject such as the management of the multiple complainer, we are dealing with an interactive process between people. Active intervention, in order to change the process, requires understanding of what is trying to be communicated, which will allow for rational correction of a distorted process, rather than simple "management" as inferred in the title. It has been amply demonstrated, whether our natural response to the complainer is a wish to keep the complainer submissive or to treat with care, that either of these approaches without real understanding usually does not bring about the alleviation of the difficulty.

It will be apparent in this discussion that the "multiple complainer" is not viewed as a clinical entity and that management must be based on understanding of the mechanisms involved. In addition, there will be no discussion of those who are complaining about realistic external or internal difficulties. Most of us accept the fact that complaints related to realistic disappointments in the performance of parents, marital partners, children, unfortunate neighbors, actions of the government and excessive demands of society are within the expectations of society. We, however, do expect that following an initial period of complaining, action will be taken by the individual to adapt to the particular situation leading to the complaints, and that a realistic solution will ensue. Likewise, complaints due to realistic disease processes or personal failures are within the cultural norm. Again, however, we expect the individual to find a more productive role for himself within a reasonable length of time. In the case of fatal and painful illness, we accept the complaints as realistic. Therefore, the group of "multiple complainers" to which we are addressing ourselves are those who are complaining but whose complaints seem to us irrational; they just complain. Clearly, then, we may react to the multiple complainer as though there is no rational explanation for his behavior. If we feel that the complaints are irrational, our reaction and our attempts to deal with the complainer are likely to be equally irrational. The solution to both sides of this interaction lies in the extension of our understanding beyond the borders of the usually acceptable reasons for "complaining" to a broader and deeper elucidation of the meaning and usefulness of the process of complaining. Increased understanding will inevitably lead to more effective management.

FORMS OF COMPLAINT

If we turn our attention for a moment to the newborn infant, we accept the fact that the infant's crying is a complaint. We realize that the cry is a form of communication—the only one available at the moment to the infant—indicating a disturbance in homeostasis, physiologic equilibrium. Through our understanding of the meaning of this complaint we are able to satisfy realistically the needs of this child in terms of water, glucose, amino acids, etc., and the complaint stops. The infant is not conscious of the specific need for water, or amino acids, or glucose, and, in fact, with the exception of water never throughout his lifetime can be conscious of the specific need for these chemicals. What is felt is a physico-chemical disequilibrium in terms of feelings of unpleasure which are communicated in a cry. From this simple model we can follow the child and its development, and recognize, as Anna Freud has pointed out, that the child does not have just a single cry but different cries to express different needs. Within a short time the mother and child unit, if not distorted by complications in the mother, the child or the environment, are able to communicate one with the other in terms of many needs. The need for alimentary and metabolic gratification is communicated, as well as the need for contact, for mouth and skin pleasure, warmth and attention. In an uncomplicated situation this to-and-fro communication leads to an orderly development of the child and of its relationships with people around it, and a pleasurable interchange between all concerned. When, however, the complaint is misunderstood, and the communication is received and misinterpreted or distorted, the need is not met, tension builds up within the child and may reach the proportions of excitement and motor activity which we, later in life, call rage, or which may reveal itself in violent disorganized motor expression similar to a temper tantrum. For example, the mother who because of excessive preoccupations of her own is unable to perceive the differences in the needs communicated by the child, and gratifies all communications by feeding, creates a situation in the infant which associates specific need with the expectation of not being gratified and of being forced to take some substitute for the specific need. The excitement (rage) which can result from this recurrent situation may intensify the mother's lack of understanding, increase her irritation at her own failure, and establish a spiraling, vicious circle.

If we follow this child from infancy through the various stages of development to adulthood and old age, we are able to take into consideration the instinctual pressures of the developing organism in their interactions with the external world. This permits us to understand the technics and solutions (character traits) which precipitate out in each individual, and with which he attempts to find the most successful solution available in the unavoidable conflicts of growth. These precipitates additively determine what we commonly call personality. The less the needs of the developing organism are understood, the more they may be met in an irrational and distorted manner. One or more of these distortions and substitutes may become the leit-motif of that individual's way of life, and as technics fixed in the personality are destined to fail even further in their need-filling purpose. It is necessary, therefore, in the management of the multiple complainer, to understand the meaning of the communication which is inherent in the complaint. To do this requires an accurate understanding of the process being observed and its genesis, or, in other words, a *total diagnosis*.

FINDING THE CAUSE

It is now common knowledge and practice when faced with a problem of multiple complaints in any individual, if the complaints are physical, to perform a careful medical history, physical examination and all of the essential laboratory studies. We have learned that it is essential to believe in our technics of examination, and to accept the positive or negative evidence that they reveal even though they throw no light upon the complaints of the individual. Likewise, if the complaints are not physical but have to do with complaints about people, we carefully examine the external situation. Thorough discussion with others who are familiar with the details of the social problem being complained about may yield a more objective view of the situation. If the complaint is about feelings which are largely subjective the neurologic apparatus is examined to rule out difficulties in perception and evaluation. Once these studies are done and no "realistic" explanation is forthcoming for either the physical, social, or subjective feeling complaints, our *total diagnosis* must continue. To return to the definition given earlier of *complain* we must try to understand what the complainer is attempting to say when he *gives utterance to grief, pain, discontent,* and, secondly, to find out against whom and toward whom they *make* this *complaint or charge.*

If one is familiar with the anatomy, the physiology and the pathology of the psyche, or, in other words, understands the factors involved in personality development from infancy to death, and gives the complainer an opportunity to communicate in these terms it is often possible rather quickly to arrive at an understanding of what the patient is trying to say, and, in a sense, to whom he is trying to say it. Our goal is to understand not the actual complaint that is being expressed, but that for which it is a substitute, the mechanism that is being used, and the need being expressed. In a sense then, we, as physicians attempting to help the multiple complainer, must endeavor to understand the communications; to set up a situation in which this communication can take place; and once understood to assist in learning new technics which will permit realistic gratification for the complainer.

There are patients with multiple complaints in whom no evidence of physical abnormality can be found, and who are often referred to as neurasthenics or hypochondriacs. These are not clinical entities and represent only a small fraction of those who should be included among the "multiple complainers." Actually, patients who have chronic physiologic disorders, which may or may not lead to structural change of the body, are also complaining even though not in a verbal sense. The concomitant physiologic hyperactivity or hypoactivity associated with an emotional state resulting from the difficulty of expressing and receiving gratification because of distortions in personality development mentioned above are actually complaints. These disturbances are primary or basic processes whose reverberations we usually only hear as secondary complaints about the pain or discomfort. We are all familiar with the pseudo gratification that may be obtained by the patient through attention and treatment of these secondary complaints, and are equally familiar with the fact that treatment in these terms usually has no lasting effectiveness. Similarly, behavior problems in children, and in adults, as well as the neuroses and the psychoses, are in reality forms of complaint. These clinical states represent attempts at solution and of gratification of various needs to which that individual has resorted as the only apparent solution available at the time. Obviously, then, the multiple complainer includes the entire gamut of maladaptation and requires an understanding of these mechanisms if definitive etiologically valid diagnosis and treatment is to be obtained. We now know and can see that multiple complaints, even if they are only in terms of verbal complaints (neurasthenia, hypochondriasis), represent merely a form of communication which the patient is attempting, and may be related to any of the more specific psychiatric syndromes. Thus, the multiple complainer may be masking a more serious disturbance, such as schizophrenia, and attempting to remain integrated through the contact obtained from the secondary gain resulting from his complaints. Again, the verbal preoccupation of the patient with the whole or a part of the body may be the outcroppings of an underlying depressive process. Frequently an underlying phobia may be masked by the discussion with the doctor of various disease processes. We would be in gross error, therefore, if we were to assume that there was an entity known as the multiple complainer and that there was a specific treatment for this entity. If the complaints are looked on as symptoms of an underlying disturbed process of adaptation and as methods of communication, no matter how unrealistic and distorted they may seem, we can be led to an understanding of the mechanism involved, and through this to the application of technics of treatment.

EXAMPLES OF DIAGNOSIS AND TREATMENT

Two case examples may be useful.

A 43-year-old, white, doctor's wife was referred as a barbiturate addict because she would not refrain from taking Nembutal and Seconal which she stole from her husband's medical bag. Her history revealed that for the past several years she had felt increasing fatigue and inability to perform her housework, had withdrawn from active participation in community affairs in which she had been a leader, and had complained of numerous physical and emotional disturbances for which she was studied by various medical specialists with unremarkable findings. Continuing complaints about pelvic discomfort, however, did lead to the performance of a hysterectomy which was followed by the excessive use of alcohol followed by the gradual beginning of the taking of barbiturates. As a result of the rather chronic confusion produced by chronic barbiturate use, she had become socially embarrassing to her physician husband and to his practice, and was increasingly avoided by her friends. As informant, the distraught husband, "at the end of his rope," revealed his anger and irritation by his facial expression and inflection as he described the situation, despite the fact that his words belied this feeling. This was further revealed by his almost complete avoidance of the patient while she was in the hospital. Thus one side of this interpersonal disequilibrium could be gauged quantitatively.

After several days of reduction and withdrawal of the drugs, an interview without interruptions was arranged to attempt to understand the process in the patient. Before this interview took place, careful evaluation of the multiple somatic complaints was completed as rapidly as possible, and occasional short "social" visits were made to the patient. When it was clear that no organic nor major physiologic disturbance was present, it was possible to approach the problem having definitely removed these factors as contributing. When it was clear early in the interview that the doctor had set aside a length of time for protracted discussion without interruptions, she began to exhibit ingratiating and somewhat seductive social graces which were helpful in understanding her "communication." She responded to the doctor's "Well?" with a recital of complaints of a physical nature. When she had been told in a kindly but firm way that there was no evidence of any major organic or physiologic disturbance, and that no further studies need be done in this regard, but that her complaints were real and we wished to understand the meaning of them and how they might be ways of expressing something which she hadn't had an opportunity to talk about, she launched into a story of her life with gradually increasing emotional coloring. In essence, she had been the only girl in a group of three siblings of moderately well-to-do parents. Her gestation, delivery and neonatal period were without major disturbance. As she approached the age of three to six, her father showered increasing attention upon her to the point of indulgence. The patient remembered in association to this discussion that she had felt that there was, at this time, dissension between her mother and the father. She stated, when asked if she had any idea of its cause, that she felt that mother thought that father was paying her (the patient) too much attention, "spoiling" her. The patient felt that the only way in which she could feel close to her mother during this time and afterwards was when she was ill, at which times mother was very solicitous in her care and interest. The patient spontaneously reflected that she must have learned to use this technic almost consciously. During her adolescence she was physically attractive, and being a member of a prominent family, was the object of much attention by many boys. Despite her success as a good student, she was able to have a great deal of satisfying social activity. This led to a bilaterally satisfying marriage around 20, with only a temporary problem in regard to her sexual relationship with her husband. She was happy and pleased to be the wife of a physician which made her prominent in the community and brought her a great deal of social attention. This was rewarded by her husband's praise for helping him in his career. Over the next few years she had several children, all of them boys, on whom she showered a great deal of attention and care, and who returned it to her in a manner which was very gratifying to her. In order to obtain a level of education which this patient and her husband felt was indicated, it was decided that the boys should go away to a private boarding school at the time of high school. They all subsequently went on to college. This gradually removed from the home all of the sons except at the usual vacation periods. In fact as the patient saw it, it was "the end of having any sons." She felt once they had left for boarding school that she really never had them again. They all developed interests in other people and girls and places and even though they were at home for a few days at vacation time, spent their summers and other vacations in active social events or in jobs elsewhere in the state or out of the state. Simultaneously she developed a feeling that her husband no longer cared for her. She felt that he was "wedded" to his large and busy practice. She then recalled how she had begun to test her husband's interest in her in almost direct proportion to her feeling of neglect by her sons. She began having various types of physical complaints which required her withdrawing from her social and civic activities and demanded medication and treatment of her husband. He referred her to colleagues for evaluation and became increasingly disturbed as the complaints increased in number with no findings. He became irritated at her and she in turn was even more convinced of his lack of interest. She tried in several of these spells of multiple complaints to return home to mother, and after an initial period of relief, found that her symptoms increased in intensity, as she saw it "because Daddy was gone and Mother had more complaints than I did." Aside from occasional flashes of understanding of this situation, the failure of communication between these two people increased. Following her hysterectomy, which she stated "ended all hope for me as a woman and made me into a useless nothing," she began to take occasional drinks of sherry during the day. As her drinking became obvious to her husband, he became quite angry and adamant in his requirement that no alcoholic beverages be kept in the house and that she was not to drink anywhere else. Since it was usual to have drinks at social occasions, this led to increasing acrimony between the two. As a substitute, she began to steal barbiturates from his bag since she had found in the past that this had given her relief. She carried this to the point where she was in a chronic state of barbiturate toxication, leading to her hospitalization. She stated, "He finally got rid of me." She actually had the feeling that he felt that she was "gone" for good. Throughout this entire discourse which lasted about an hour and a half, very few direct questions were asked. Communication from the interviewer to the patient was largely in the sense of head nodding in the affirmative, facial expressions to indicate understanding of the feelings associated with what was being said, expectant waiting during periods of silence, as well as indications to the patient that the things she was talking about were rational and realistic and part of a life process. At this point in the interview, the patient had returned to the present and to the precipitating situation. The amount of feeling that was associated with the description that she had given had brought her to the point of tears and a statement regarding the hopelessness of her situation. The interviewer indicated verbally his understanding of the situation and suggested that perhaps it would be easier to think about this overnight and talk about it again the next day. The patient, who was weeping at this time, agreed. The interview was terminated after a few minutes of reassurance that things did not look so hopeless and that there unquestionably was a way out.

On the following day the patient obviously brightened and was prepared for the interviewer in the sense of having fixed her hair and her face and her clothing, but began by apologizing for her behavior yesterday. The interviewer then recapitulated what had been said the day before by the patient and his understanding of her feeling of gradually being "not needed by anyone" and "that nobody cared" and that she was now "useless." He compared this with her feelings of pleasure at the attention of her father, then of her sons, and then of her husband, and how illness and sickness had been the way that she had related to her mother in the past. She rather quickly made the jump in time and was able to see in part how her present behavior could be a recapitulation of the way she had related in the past when she felt that she wasn't getting the attention she wanted and that the technics were similar. She stated that in thinking over what had happened in the previous interview she suddenly had the feeling that when the interviewer came the next day, she would just like to sit in his lap and put her head on his shoulder and cry. The interviewer responded to this with a statement of understanding, but asking the patient to consider how long she thought that this would be pleasing to her, and that if actually she hadn't in a sense been coddling herself this way as she wanted her mother to do long ago and had been wanting her husband and other doctors to do for the past several years. After an initial rather intense rage reaction toward the interviewer whom she claimed was "cold and hard," she stated, "You are the first one who has ever actually made me look at myself. The others just got angry, did another test, and I either left immediately or finally realized nothing was coming of it all. I can see that I am really acting in a pouting, demanding way and that there isn't much future in this." This led her to a discussion, with evidence of some pleasure, of how active she had been in community affairs when her boys had been home. She admitted that the civic demands and requests for her particular leadership were now even stronger than they had been previously, yet she had been unable to take on any of them. She realized that she had been only a detriment to her husband and to his practice in terms of his worry about her, her demands upon him, and her embarrassment of him socially. At the end of this interview she stated, "There is no percentage in this. I realize now that I can't just expect to be loved in the way I was as a little child, but I have to deserve to be loved. My sons haven't deserted me; they have grown up. They haven't stopped loving me, but I can't expect them to love me to the exclusion of everyone else and I have really neglected my husband for a number of years as my boys and outside activities filled my time. I don't need you any more; I am not crazy, and I want to get out of here." She accepted the suggestion that she rest overnight and review the situation the next day. The third interview was in a sense a recapitulation by the patient of her under-standing of the situation and her realization that for her to have the attention and interest of other people, she would have to give some-thing to them as she had previously done. It was decided to ask the husband to join in the discussion and the entire matter was rehashed. This led to a realization on his part of a feeling that she had not been interested in him in the past as she showed attention to the boys. He had responded with an increasing withdrawal into his work.

These two people, after the verbalization of what were understandable human reactions based on our knowledge of human needs and developmental principles, were able to communicate with each other in real terms for the first time in many years. The result was the return home of the patient and her husband to a much more realistic and obvious interest in each other. The patient now writes on the anniversary of her hospital visit and at Christmas that she is reasonably happy, that she is busily engaged in a number of civic activities of interest to her, and that two of her sons are married, and that she is having a great deal of pleasure in occasionally seeing them and helping them in financial and other needs. Although the illness, and the difficulty in communicating had been serious, the relative soundness of her personality made it possible for her to gain insight into the unreality of her complaints, her distorted attempt at communicating, and, once seen, to begin to gratify her needs in a more realistic and mature manner. She no longer required alcohol, barbiturates and other expressions of anger as her way of seeking understanding and fulfillment.

This patient could easily have been diagnosed as involutional, alcoholic, addiction reaction, hypochondriac, neurasthenic, neurotic or spoiled woman. Treatment of any of these diagnoses instead of the process had failed for several years. Treatment based on understanding the present meaning of her attempts to communicate her needs and their past derivatives was quickly and permanently successful.

In contrast is another patient who was "managed" by Dr. Charles Vernon of our department, and who shows the results of lifelong distortion in communication and the gratification of needs. Real deprivation led to serious distortion in her attempt to obtain attention from her father. The complexity of this situation, its understanding and management are described below.

When this 16-year-old white, single girl with diabetes was transferred to the psychiatric ward she had become an intolerable management problem for the personnel on the medical ward, and, as one interne wrote in the chart (and this was the chief complaint of the doctors who referred her to psychiatry), "She is never without some complaint."

She had been referred to the medical service in April, 1953, in a severe state of malnutrition from anorexia and diabetic acidosis. By history it was certain her diabetes mellitus had gone for at least two years untreated although diagnosed. Also, on admission, it was ascertained that she had an acute pyelonephritis and severely carious teeth, all evidence of real but avoidable deprivation. She responded well to medical treatment of the diabetes and the infection, and immediately began engorging large quantities of food, even over and above the final 5,000 calorie diet they were eventually felt forced to put her on, gaining weight in the first two weeks from 90 to 100 pounds. After about three weeks of gradual improvement, it was decided that all her teeth should be extracted, and this was accomplished over a period of about one week in the latter part of May. She received minimal preparation for this procedure other than her consent to have it carried out, although from the reports of the personnel at the time she seemed willing enough to have this done and understood the necessity for it. Later it became clear that the extractions meant a great deal more to her than was understood at the time either by her, consciously, or by her attending physicians. Her pleasure in eating (being loved and given to) had not been understood and her extractions were reacted to again as painful deprivation.

It was during these dental procedures that she developed numerous complaints, most notably abdominal pain and anorexia. This was followed by the discovery during the succeeding two weeks of a huge stomach ulcer, vascular hypertension (160 over 120), unexplained eosinophilia, calcific pancreatitis and peripheral neuropathy. The response to these organ "complaints" was more and more medical investigation and manipulation with all the various ingenious devices for exploring the orifices. Each new symptom or sign (e.g., intermittent diarrhea, rectal bleeding, chest pain) was met with further physical tests and re-evaluations and continued frustration of both patient and doctor. Some 60-odd diagnostic procedures were done during the period between her dental extractions and admission to psychiatry. These included repeated examinations of blood, urine and feces, and repeated diagnostic procedures such as x-rays, anoscopic exams, pancreatic studies, etc. Analgesics, sedation and placebos gave equivocal results so far as her abdominal pain was concerned; the most consistently effective analgesic was actually *any medication* given by injection.

Her constant demanding attitude, the developing difficulties in getting her to eat, and the apparently intractable pain led to calling for psychiatric consultation four weeks after the dental extractions, and finally, in desperation, transfer to the psychiatric ward was effected one month later in early August. By this time her weight was down to 80 pounds, and it was felt that death was imminent if something were not done.

On the psychiatric service she was seen in daily interviews by the resident assigned to her case. All complaints and problems were directed by the nurses, aides and other ward personnel to this one physician, who had sole responsibility for her care. Medications except insulin and pancreatin were stopped (after a trial of heavy barbiturate sedation to no avail) , and she was put on a liberal diabetic diet. A firm, consistent, nonpunitive, and hopefully realistic attitude was maintained, or at least aimed for, by all personnel. A stormy period of four to six weeks followed during which time she began to verbalize and act out directly terrific hostility toward the therapist and ward personnel. Her verbal tirades about the therapist were put in the same manner as she had previously described her father's brutality to her. This culminated by her leaving the hospital, for a brief time, without permission in October. It was quite obvious that she expected to be beaten as she had been by her father for this behavior. When this was not forthcoming she at first did not know how to "communicate" or get along with her therapist and only after some weeks did she find ways of gratifying her need for attention in less complex and traumatic manner. After this she gradually stopped complaining of pain, became normotensive, gained weight, and roentgenograms revealed that her stomach ulcer was healed. The pyelonephritis had been taken care of effectively before transfer. She was eventually discharged in November of that year, four months after transfer, in a remarkably changed state of mind and body, and in a positive, fatherlike relationship with the therapist. Outpatient follow-up has been effective now with a regular visit, usually monthly, to the clinic. Continued improvement has been maintained although major and minor setbacks have occurred to date (December 1955) .

How she became so tragically involved with all personnel after entering the hospital is the pertinent problem, and raises many questions. She was admitted to the hospital truly physically ill with a number of so-called diagnostic entities for which there are well defined and accepted therapies. All those (medical student, interne and resident) who took histories on admission accurately noted the difficulties she had had with her diabetic father (a night watchman) who was physically brutal toward her and intolerant of her illness and who considered her progressive weakness preceding hospitalization as dilatoriness and laziness. Further it was well recorded that she had had repeated episodes of abdominal pain since adolescence with various diagnoses offered, and that her main difficulties had begun since an appendectomy in puberty (actually at age ten), at which time she began to lose weight, having been markedly obese up until this time (i.e., weight 150 pounds) . The mother reported also later that her behavioral difficulties had really begun and become "bad" after this appendectomy. It was also revealed that she had been relatively deprived and had to scramble for food, as well as for psychological gratifications, all her life since leaving the breast at age one. She had three older siblings and two younger ones and provisions were always short. Even at the age of one she was diagnosed as having rickets (a physiologic deprivation of vitamins) and required treatment with cod liver oil.

Of course, it is quite easy in retrospect to criticize the handling of this patient and to wonder if it should not have been predicted that trouble would occur following as traumatic a procedure as extractions of teeth in the light of her past difficulties. And further, should one not have expected her to react to the hospital authorities after such a traumatic procedure similarly to the way she reacted in the past toward her father? Had these retrospectively obvious factors been recognized at the time, the question arises, "Could anything have been done about it by a different approach, assuming probably quite correctly that her teeth should have been extracted for sound medical reasons. Considering the success of the total therapeutic endeavor on the psychiatric ward, it would seem that probably something could have been done. Following this through, the question then arises, "What are the essential differences in these two approaches?", the one on the medical ward and the one on the psychiatric ward?

One way of approaching this without going into the more complicated processes involved would be to say that for a variety of reasons the total diagnosis was missed in this case, and while numerous laboratory procedures were being carried out, the indicated investigative procedure of the meaning and genesis of the process was not properly, or to its full advantage, utilized. The patient was expressing through her organs in the only way she knew (at least under stress) her difficulties and distorted methods of communicating her needs in interpersonal relationships. Interpersonal distress, therefore, was being expressed implicitly by physiologic disturbance. No lasting or effective alleviation of this distress could be expected without appreciation of this process.

The patient did not acquire any intellectual insight into her behavior, as did the first patient. She learned instead a new and more realistic way of communicating and gratifying her needs through her experience with her consistently kind but firm and hope-inducing therapist. Distorted methods of communicating and attempting gratification were not rewarding whereas realistic technics commensurate with her age and condition were successful. No complex formulations or psychological technics were needed or used. She learned to "live" less complexly and more pleasurably. "Complaints" of all kinds were increasingly nonproductive and "management" was, in essence, consistent friendliness.

Again treatment of "correct" medical diagnoses failed because a *total diagnosis* was not made.

Time and space do not permit the giving of other examples. Actually they are not necessary for they exhibit themselves constantly in everyday living and everyday medical practice. Patients and nonpatients have complaints that may be chronic or short-lived, multiple or few in number. They are all attempting to gratify needs and to communicate to those around them. Likewise there are those who wish to help or to "manage." It is obvious that success depends upon understanding the meaning of the complainer if we are to help him toward a more realistic fulfillment of their needs.

If we return to our dictionary definitions, it is interesting to see how, as a distillate of the wisdom and the experience of people, our language has expressed so clearly these several aspects of the problem we have just discussed.

To give utterance to grief, pain, and discontent; to strike, beat the breast in grief, or lament, expresses the depth and the intensity of the need and of the feeling of misunderstanding and the lack of gratification. The second definition, *to make formal accusation or charge,* is so clearly the frustrated rage inherent in the lack of fulfillment. The definitions of *manage* contain within them the broad gamut of human reaction to the complainer. The angry reaction inherent in the frustration of the person wishing to help but responding to the anger and resentment of the complainer is described in the definition *to render and keep one submissive.* Various other shades of attitude in the manager are evidenced in the definitions, *to control and direct;* the less dominating attitude, *to conduct, to guide and to administer,* and a still warmer attitude is evidenced in the definition *to treat with care, to husband.*

In summary, there is no distinct entity which can be called the multiple complainer, only a process. To manage or treat this process requires an understanding of the meaning and goals of the process. Since complaints are the medium of communications between patient and doctor, there are several concrete suggestions that can be made which, if followed, can be of assistance in a more successful management. They are an enlargement as well as a paraphrase of a similar statement made by Karl Menninger in "The Human Mind." These suggestions are as follows:

First, arrive at a *total diagnosis.*

Second, acquire a working knowledge of the anatomy, physiology, and pathology of personality development equal to your knowledge of the somatic development and function. Useful descriptions of these matters are available in such books as English and Pearson's "Emotional Problems of Living," and others.

Third, do not treat a diagnosis. Quickly evaluate the possibility, extent or absence of organic disturbances or physiologic disturbances, and have trust and confidence in your technics and laboratory procedures. Do not fall back on more laboratory procedures because your "management" does not seem to be producing a reduction in complaints or an improvement in the patient quickly. Once determined, be definite in your explanations to the patient about the absence of physical disturbances or the weight that should be given to any that are present.

Fourth, show the patient that you are interested in him whether or not he has a physical disturbance.

Fifth, don't lie, give placebos or joke about the symptoms, and don't promise what you're not sure you can produce.

Sixth, listen to what the patient has to say; listen a long time and frequently, alone and without interruption.

Seventh, be nonjudgmental in word and attitude. Do not rebuke, ridicule, or depreciate. An understanding of the conscious and unconscious needs of patients is the greatest deterrent to being disturbed or to laughing at what seem to be ridiculous ideas or feelings of the patient.

Eighth, don't give advice or treatment or an opinion until you know what really is wrong with the patient, and then tell him that you think that his difficulty could be (not is) related to the present and past disturbances that have been discussed.

Ninth, gradually help the patient to a realization and a connection between his complaints and his distorted technics of attempting to obtain gratification. Help him to find the connection between these factors and their derivation in the past. Help him to assume responsibility for more successful technics which will more closely approximate continued and realistic gratification of his continuing needs. This represents a rational therapy based on understanding of process and therefore etiologically oriented and offers the only permanently successful method that we have available.

THE MANAGEMENT OF OVEREATING,
OVERDRINKING AND OVERSMOKING

Leo H. Bartemeier, M.D.

In a former time every obese person was advised to lose weight. Every alcoholic was told that he must make up his mind to stop drinking, and every heavy smoker was warned to reduce his daily consumption of tobacco. Today we are more cautious regarding the management of overindulgence because we have learned that overeating, overdrinking and oversmoking are the manifestations of many different kinds of emotional problems. Food, drink and tobacco are consistently consumed in excessive quantities to satisfy a great variety of psychological needs. To recommend that everyone who eats too much should eat less and lose weight would be like recommending that everyone suffering from headaches should take aspirin. Just as it is necessary to examine each person who suffers from headaches in order to learn what causes them, so it is only intelligent to follow the same procedure with each person who overindulges in food, drink or tobacco. Overindulgence is a symptom of some disturbance of the emotional life as certainly as headache or fever or any other symptoms of illness. But unlike these affections, overeating, overdrinking and oversmoking are pleasurable and satisfying. It is this very quality that makes dieting and abstinence so difficult and so often impossible.

When people feel sick they tend to doctor themselves. They frequently do not know what ails them, but they hope it is not serious and that it will pass away. In some instances it does, but in others their symptoms persist, and not until they become frightened do they summon their physicians. Many a man who thought he was having acute indigestion was suffering from a coronary thrombosis and by the time a medical man arrived it was too late. Similarly many people have abstained from cigarette smoking because of the publicity about lung cancer, but those who eat and drink excessively have no such publicity to frighten them. No one dies from being too heavy and though everyone has heard of someone who drank himself to death no heavy drinker believes this could happen to him. It is also probable that the majority of heavy cigarette smokers have not been frightened by the cancer publicity because the evidence has not been conclusive and because filter tip advertising has been quite convincing. Also, many people have adhered to reducing diets and have overcome their obesity only to become obese again. They are impelled to overeating by inner demands over which they have no control, or which they succeed in controlling only temporarily. In other respects they manifest excellent control. That excessive consumption of food or alcohol or tobacco is connected with the emotions and that it has specific meaning and significance for each person is well known to psychiatric and psychoanalytic clinicians, to many general practitioners of medicine and to many nonprofessional people as well. Freed found that 93 per cent of 500 obese patients were aware of the relation between their eating patterns and their emotions.[1]

Brosin[2] wrote that "the physician can estimate the relative severity of the patient's conflicts in one of the four categories described by Dr. W. W. Hamburger,[3] who regarded overeating as a response to nonspecific emotional tensions; overeating as a substitute gratification in intolerable life situations; overeating as a symptom of an underlying emotional illness, especially depressions and hysteria; and overeating as an addiction to food."

Brosin went on to say that "the patients who use the mechanisms of the first two classes are relatively amenable to the treatment measures that are used by all physicians in their total care of the patient. The third class may require psychiatric consultation or, in severe cases, to be referred to a psychiatrist.—The fourth group of patients who use food as other patients use drugs are usually sick enough to require intensive psychiatric treatment.

"Psychiatric experience with obese patients shows a wide variety of conflicts and psychiatric syndromes. While many patients have some features in common, it is unsafe to generalize about common factors in the single case. Every patient is an individual whose life patterns are distinctive for him.—Most of us like to eat good food and can appreciate those satisfactions that come with a good dinner. Many well-adjusted persons know that they can improve their mood if they are discouraged about the current difficulties on a job if they have a drink and an attractive meal. Many obese persons have discovered that food acts as a sedative for them when they are anxious, downhearted, angry, disappointed, or blocked on a project. If external circumstancess improve so that the patient receives 'satisfactions' from other persons, then the need for food ingestion diminishes. This may help to explain why obesity is a self-limiting disorder in many cases and also why remarkable cures are possible when circumstances permit a favorable realignment of the patient's activities. It may also help to explain the success of social clubs formed by obese persons, modeled on Alcoholics Anonymous, because these organizations offer much companionship and realistic support from persons who have intimate appreciation of the powerful inner drives to overeat."

Doctor Brosin concluded his article with a caution to physicians "about weight-reducing programs for patients in middle life. Many of them are hard-working men and women who unfortunately receive relatively little satisfaction from their families or their jobs. These persons may be highly successful and important in their work but use intakes of various kinds to give them pleasure. If one takes away smoking, food and alcohol from such a delicately balanced person, one has the obligation to put something constructive in its place. For two years I have seen patients who hearing about cancer have stopped smoking. In some men this has resulted in considerable weight gains up to forty pounds. Now they dread the consequences of added weight. This is an example of the equivalence between one set of activities and another."

Some persons who managed their overeating successfully are known to have subsequently developed an inability to eat which then persisted for several months. Gradually they regained their appetite and their overeating returned. These persons have demonstrated that overeating and its opposite, the inability to eat, are two facets of a single process. The loss of the desire to eat and the accompanying loss of weight likewise occur in patients who suffer from depressions. Like overeating, the inability to eat also has its specific meaning and significance. In this connection it may be worth noting that the word obesity which "is derived from the

Latin *'obedere'* from *ob,* intensive, plus *edere,* to eat, has worked both ways. At first it was applied to a person eaten away, very lean; then, to one that devoured all he could, and became very fat. The fat meaning of obese has devoured the lean one."[4]

Doctor Sebrell, of the United States Public Health Service, speaking at the National Food and Nutrition Institute in 1952, said that "obesity has replaced the vitamin deficiency diseases as the number one nutrition problem in the United States. An estimated one-fourth of the adults in this country are obese—that is, sufficiently overweight to result in an appreciable damage to health; and the incidence may reach 60 per cent in older women. Experimental evidence points to the life-shortening effects of obesity."

No discussion of overeating, overdrinking and oversmoking would be complete if it did not include the social pressures which contribute to these problems. Within recent times both business and the professions have developed the custom of arranging luncheon and dinner meetings to save the time of busy persons and to increase the attendance of those who are expected to attend. Eating and drinking together makes for sociability and improves the exchange of ideas. These meetings also contribute to the development of obesity and alcoholism in those individuals who are predisposed toward these conditions. The pressure to conform to the social behavior of others in these situations is an equally important contributing factor. One who declines to drink with others in some of these gatherings is apt to draw attention to himself, to be questioned about his not drinking and to be made to feel that he is either mildly disliked or at least that he is in disfavor. There are groups in which a nondrinker may even be ridiculed or otherwise embarrassed. Subsequently, he may be excluded from the group because of his sobriety. The pressures to eat and drink all that is offered are so great that one cannot accept dinner invitations if one is determined to adhere consistently to prescribed dietary restrictions. To abstain from drinking and to eat sparingly when being entertained by friends or relatives has come to signify unfriendliness, frank impoliteness or even an insulting way to behave.

Some persons indulge in excessive smoking to obtain the satisfaction which their work does not provide them. They are like some children who insist they can study better while listening to soft radio music. Smoking, like drinking or eating, has many different meanings for different people and there are many who depend upon excessive indulgence in one form or another to avoid anxiety, to be able to work and to be friendly or sociable with others. When they eat less, smoke less or quit drinking, they become unreasonably irritable, quarrelsome and sensitive to comments by others which had previously not affected them. Others become depressed, lose interest in work and social relations, develop insomnia and think about suicide.

The self-management of these problems is not as simple a procedure as it appears. Many excessive drinkers, for example, who are known to have developed complete abstinence from alcohol have replaced their drinking with sedatives or narcotic drugs. Excessive smokers who gave up their cigarettes have often reverted to their earlier method of self-indulgence for which their smoking was originally a substitute. Overeating, overdrinking and oversmoking are minor modifications of the primary mouth satisfactions of infancy which accompany the nursing activity. In addition to the relief of hunger and thirst, the infant needs the optimum of pleasure and satisfaction of the impulses to suck, to bite and later to chew. If these gratifications are either diminished or supplied too abundantly through the influence of the mother, these instinctual impulses are thereby intensified. It is this mismanagement of the earliest mouth satisfactions which prepares the pattern for excessive eating, drinking and smoking when other emotional disturbances develop during later living. Obesity in adolescent girls, for example, like many instances of colic in infants, is frequently found to be a manifestation of a long history of emotional dissatisfaction in their relations with their mothers and their fathers. It is useless to expect that such problems as these can be corrected by dieting when it is so apparent that the excessive appetite and eating of these girls are but other forms of hunger for love and being loved by their mothers and fathers. Simultaneously, their obesity is usually more displeasing to their parents than it is to themselves. Their inability to reduce their weight is a manifestation of the continuing revenge as well as the emotional satisfaction they derive from their excessive eating. The successful management of such patients has been achieved most frequently through the persistent kindness and understanding of family physicians and specialists in the field of mental health. The diminution of both the appetite and the need for excessive eating has been replaced by the quality of the relationship between the patient and the physician.

The management of prolonged and excessive drinking is exceedingly difficult and oftentimes impossible. This is especially true with persons who are 50 and past. Those who are chronically alcoholic, like those who are addicted to narcotic drugs, are usually disinclined to seek treatment for themselves from physicians in the general practice of medicine or from psychiatrists or even to turn for advice from their own religious leaders. It is this lack of motivation which is outstanding and which often leaves one with the impression that they are bent on their own self-destruction. Most of them are quite aware of the unhappiness they bring to their families and although they seem sincere in their resolutions to discontinue their drinking, they rarely are able to carry them out for any reasonable period of time. They behave as though their alcoholism protects them from something within themselves of which they are terrified. They remind one to some extent of other persons who, sensing a vague awareness that they are hopelessly ill because of cancer, decide to commit suicide. The victims of chronic alcoholism undoubtedly carry out a slow and prolonged suicidal process. As Karl Menninger says, "the alcoholic suffers secretly from unspeakable terror which he cannot bear to face. He knows only the device of drowning the fear by drinking and his 'cure' (drinking) then becomes worse than the disease, at least so far as outside evidences are concerned.—The victim of alcohol addiction knows what most of his critics do not know, namely, that alcoholism is not a disease, or at least not the principal disease from which he suffers; furthermore, he knows that he does not know the origin or nature of the dreadful pain and fear within him which impel him, blindly, to alcoholic self-destruction. It is like some poor beast who has been poisoned or set on fire and runs blindly into the sea to court one death in fleeing another.

"Indeed, we frequently see patients who start out with conscious suicidal intuitions and end up by getting drunk (or who get drunk first in order to make a suicidal attempt), as if his was (or it is) a less certain death than shooting. Many of the patients treated for alcoholic addiction are preoccupied in their sober moments with thoughts of self-destruction, sometimes coupled with realization of their own unworthiness, sinfulness, and incompetence.— Thus alcohol addiction can be thought of not as a disease, but as a suicidal flight from disease, a disastrous attempt at the self-cure of an unseen inner conflict, aggravated but not primarily caused (as many think) by external conflict. It is literally true that the alcoholic, as he himself says, does not know why he drinks."[5]

Excessive drinkers and those who are addicted to alcohol are persons whose emotional development has been damaged very early in their lives. They may give the impression of being healthy and they often appear to be charming and very sociable. Beneath this outer façade, however, they are lonely and are lacking any genuine feeling for other persons. The mismanagement of their basic needs during their infancy has predisposed them to their later alcoholism.

A 43-year-old clergyman of good intelligence, who occasionally had engaged in a moderate amount of social drinking, had seemingly fulfilled his obligations toward his parishioners quite satisfactorily. He was, however, obviously unable to withstand his separation from his mother which was occasioned by her death. Quite soon after he had suffered her loss he began to indulge in solitary drinking in his room. His drinking became so steady and so excessive that he could no longer perform his clerical functions. His solitary drinking was the replacement of his earliest relation with his mother. When deprived of alcohol through his admission to a hospital he became depressed and spoke of wanting to die so that he might be re-united with his mother.

A 52-year-old married woman who often experienced a strong impulse to murder her husband would frequently render herself unconscious with large quantities of alcohol. She drank whenever she became aware of her homicidal feeling. The provocations by her husband were no more serious than those which would arouse any woman's anger. This woman's repeated periods of severe alcoholic intoxication were transitory suicidal episodes. Like many another impulsive drinker who could not tolerate frustration nor manage her destructive feelings in a more satisfactory way she turned her destructiveness against herself.

One man lost his job but soon found another and his life continued as before. Another man lost his job and instead of becoming depressed he began to drink excessively. On examination it was found that it was not the loss of the job itself but the loss of his relation with his foreman which provided him with satisfactions that were of special significance to him. When he was forced into a hospital where he no longer had access to alcohol he soon became depressed and suicidal. It was this severe emotional illness from which his alcoholism had protected him. He and his foreman had sometimes been drunk together.

The frequency of these problems in the general population is evidence of the dissatisfaction which so many people experience in their life situations. Overindulgence develops insidiously and without awareness of the dangers involved in the excessive consumption of food, alcohol and tobacco. These dangers include the slow and nonperceivable damage to the heart, the blood vessels, the brain and the liver. The easy availability of food, alcohol and tobacco, together with the social customs and pressures associated with eating and drinking, are some of the external factors which contribute to these conditions. They are, however, only secondary and of far less importance than the internal personal factors which are both psychological and physiologic, and peculiar to each individual.

It is significant that excessive eating, drinking and smoking are particularly apt to develop at the time of life when human responsibility is at its zenith. At this period people are less active and more inclined to be sedentary. Fatigue from work is more likely because work has assumed greater importance. One thinks of promotions with increased responsibilities as one example among many. Extra food, drink and tobacco provide extra fuel and additional stimulation. They relieve tension and afford protection from anxiety for a great many people. They are pleasurable and temporarily satisfying. At the same time they are self-destructive processes and most unfortunately it is this destructive aspect of overindulgence which is usually not detected until irreversible changes have taken place in vital organs and systems and the life expectancy is considerably shortened.

In the light of our present knowledge about the emotional and physiologic aspects of excessive eating, drinking and smoking, the familiar self-management of these problems now appears unwise and may also prove to be a dangerous procedure. The more intelligent course to pursue is to seek the services of a physician. Having done so it is imperative that both patient and doctor need to work together in complete sincerity and honesty with each other. They need to be prepared for failure and disappointment. They also need to know in advance that the management of these conditions is likely to be a slow and tedious process and that the necessary changes cannot be accomplished without considerable struggle.

There is general need for the more natural management of the basic emotional needs of infants. This is developing slowly but in the face of tremendous resistance to the re-establishment of practices that were in vogue in this country some 50 years ago.

There is great need for the development of new technics in public education concerning these problems. It is also certain that American medicine alone cannot succeed in the management of this problem until public interest and participation have been developed sufficiently. None of the great epidemics has been conquered by medicine alone and the same is true with regard to overeating, overdrinking and oversmoking, which foreshorten the lives of so many.

BIBLIOGRAPHY

1. Freed, S. C.: Psychic factors in development and treatment of obesity, J.A.M.A. **133**:369-373, 1947.
2. Brosin, Henry W.: The psychiatric aspects of obesity, J.A.M.A. **155**: 1238-1239, 1954.
3. Hamburger, W. W.: Emotional aspects of obesity, Med. Clin. North America 35:483-499, 1951.
4. Shipley, J. T.: Dictionary of Word Origins, Ames, Iowa, Littleford-Adams, 1955, p. 190.
5. Menninger, Karl A.: Love Against Hate, New York, Harcourt Brace, 1938, p. 160.

ON AVOIDING THE PRODUCTION OF
IATROGENIC DISEASE

Walter C. Alvarez, M.D

First, some may ask, "What is iatrogenic disease?" And the answer is: disease produced by a physician, or one of his assistants or nurses, or a druggist. The next question is, "Is such disease common?" The answer, unfortunately, must be "Yes." Even the wisest and most wary and thoughtful of us physicians must often be producing some iatrogenic anxiety, if not a long-lasting and serious neurosis which later is hard to dispel.

Unless the physician is optimistic by nature, usually correct in his diagnoses and prognoses, courageous and willing to assume the full responsibility that goes with telling a patient that he is well and safe and has nothing to worry about, and unless he is always guarded in his speech, he will occasionally frighten a patient or confuse him, or cause him much anxiety. He may even throw him into a depression, or a neurosis.

I admit that after 50 years of trying to learn to guard my tongue and to avoid saying anything that will needlessly worry my patients, every so often I learn that I have said the wrong thing and have frightened someone badly.

Problems that arise in taking the history. Sometimes the physician can wreck a patient's nervous system just by asking a foolish question. For instance: a pediatrician, called to see a child with canker sores in his mouth, asked the mother if she had ever had syphilis. This shocked her so badly that for the next two years she was in a serious depression. The young physician had made two mistakes: one, in confusing simple canker sores with mucous plaques; the second, in not recognizing that the mother was a mildly psychotic person who could not stand much in the way of worry. She could not face the idea that she and her child might have syphilis.

A hundred times I have been made a bit distressed when, in a clinic record, I have seen the usual statement of an assistant to the effect that a fine, gray-haired mother of four, "denied she had syphilis." He should not have asked such a question; he should have been satisfied with the negative report of a routine Wassermann test.

A point which I would emphasize here is that the wise physician, as he takes a history, should always be watching the person's face to note when he has touched upon a painful subject, or when he has caused the person to show dislike or anxiety or annoyance or boredom.

Every physician must constantly be guarding his tongue. It would seem obvious that all good and kindly and thoughtful physicians must constantly be guarding their tongue, especially when dealing with the type of patient who seems to crave a bad diagnosis and prognosis. We physicians must guard our tongue if only to save ourselves from the endless trouble and annoyance that can follow on a bad remark.

For instance, one day in a misguided moment, I let an anxious woman with an occasional slight diarrhea know that my bacteriologist had found in her stools a certain streptococcus (which, at that time, was supposed by some men to cause chronic ulcerative colitis). I emphasized to her the fact that most physicians had not yet accepted this streptococcus as the cause of colitis, and I advised her not to worry about it. But in the next 15 years, I had to spend many hours trying to reassure her, to cheer her up, and to undo the mental damage I had done.

One must not think aloud during the examination. One of the worst habits that some of us physicians get into is that of thinking aloud as we try to work our way to a diagnosis. Let us say that in comes a woman who tells us that for ten days she had a sort of cold, or what she thought was a cold. After that, for a month, she felt below par and occasionally a little feverish.

On examining her, the physician finds, perhaps, that she has a number of enlarged lymph nodes in her neck. If he is inexperienced and thoughtless, he may start telling her of all the awful things that such an enlargement could indicate. He might tell her about leukemia, Hodgkin's disease, bronchial cancer, or metastases from a meningioma inside her skull. As a result of this, a few days later, when he tells her that he hasn't found anything wrong, she may go away still much frightened and unhappy because she is not satisfied that he ruled out adequately all these horrible diseases.

The wise physician will say nothing but will have her blood studied to see if it contains the heterophile antibody, indicating mononucleosis. He will have a white blood count made, and the leukocytes checked to make sure the woman hasn't a leukemia. He will have an estimate made of the red blood sedimentation rate to rule out serious disease; he will have a roentgenologic study made of her thorax to rule out masses which would suggest a tumor. In the end, he may conclude that the woman is one of those many persons who, with a cold, can get large lymph nodes. Then, when he finishes his examination and tells her that there is nothing seriously wrong, she will not be worried but will go home happy.

The dangers of saying too much to a mildly psychotic person. One of the things we physicians need to do is to recognize the mildly psychotic or markedly hypochondriacal type of person to whom we had better not say much. For instance, a mildly psychotic patient who had got the idea that he might have a gastritis, went to a gastroscopist who, not recognizing the bad mental state of the man, examined him. Unfortunately, he talked as he showed his assistant the little bleeding point where the rubber tip of the instrument had scratched the mucosa. This sent the patient into a panic. He felt so sure that he had a bad ulcer that he went on a diet of nothing but milk, and remained on this until he was skin and bones. I then had a hard time talking him out of his "ulcer."

Unwise remarks made during the examination by interns, nurses or assistant physicians. Around a big hospital it is so necessary that the assistants, interns, laboratory girls, assistant roentgenologists and others be taught to say nothing around the patients. Even whispering can be dangerous because it can throw a paranoid patient into a state of suspicion.

I remember a psychotic young man who came to me with the conviction that he had a cancer of the stomach. After being roentgenoscoped, he came back, wringing his hands and weeping. He said that the roentgenologist had told him he had a hopeless cancer. Knowing that the roentgenologist would not have said anything, I asked, "Just exactly what *did* he say?" And the man replied, "He said to his assistant 'N.P.' or 'No possible hope.'" I smiled because, in that particular roentgenologic department, "N.P." was slang for "no plates"; in other words, the roentgenologist was so satisfied from his fluoroscopic examination that the stomach was normal that he did not want a lot of films made.

I remember another young man who, while suffering an ordinary nosebleed, was terribly frightened by an intern's remark that the cause might well be an acute leukemia which could lead to a hemorrhage into the brain! This information threw the man into such a panic that I doubt if I succeeded later in straightening him out.

Nurses can, at times, put painful ideas into a patient's head. I have known a nurse to say to a woman who had just come into a hospital for an operation, "You know, the woman who this morning died in your bed there had the same operation you are going to have and she was dead in two days!" Another nurse wrecked the mental peace of one of my patients by telling her that her herpes zoster was probably due to syphilis!

Another woman was mentally upset for several years by a druggist's statement that a little potassium iodide I had given her for her asthma was usually prescribed for syphilis.

A woman of culture who, through a tactless remark, had been given the idea by her physician that she might have syphilis, spent a year getting repeated Wassermann tests. Because all were negative, she had begun to feel reassured, when another physician said to her, so cruelly, "But you know that a negative Wassermann is not absolute proof that you haven't syphilis." After this, there was no consoling the poor woman, and never again did she feel clean.

Problems that arise in reporting insignificant findings. Most iatrogenic diseases are produced as we physicians report to the patient what we found. Some of the problems of what to say and not to say are so difficult that I have never been able to solve them to my satisfaction. Let us say that, while going over a nervous woman with no symptoms to indicate organic disease, I find a slight heart murmur, or a silent bundle branch block, or a little increase in blood pressure, or a silent cervical rib, or a small harmless diaphragmatic hernia, or a cholesterol stone floating around in a normally functioning and silent gallbladder, or some harmless diverticula on the colon, or a partial failure of rotation of the colon, or a striking ptosis of the stomach. I would much prefer not to mention these things and I may dread to mention them, especially to a hypochondriacal type of patient. Mentioning them can only do harm.

But there is a difficulty. If I do not mention them, at the patient's next medical overhauling, they will again be found, and then, if the doctor mentions them to the patient, and especially if he looks on them as the cause of the symptoms "which I missed," my standing with that patient will become very low. He (or she) may well think that I was incompetent or that I made an inexpert examination. Often I take the risk to my reputation and make no mention of the findings. When I do feel that I must mention something I emphasize to the patient, and, if possible, to his relatives, that it means nothing or nothing important, and it must not be treated. It is not producing the symptoms, and it will not bring the patient to any bad end.

In spite of all this, time and again I have later heard that the patient with, let us say, a perfectly silent and harmless gallstone went straight to a surgeon and insisted on having it out.

One of my failures. I was humbled one day when I saw a woman whom, years before, I had got out of an unnecessary wheel chair and restored to health. During several interviews I had tried to get her to see how, after years of overwork, strain, unhappiness and undisciplined and unhygienic living, her nerves had got to playing miserable tricks on her. What later surprised and distressed me was to hear her say that for years she had lived in terror because I had left her with the idea that the paralysis would soon return and become incurable!

The great need for saying nothing about minor changes in roentgenograms and laboratory reports. One of the unfortunate things many of us physicians commonly do is to take the roentgenograms of a highly neurotic woman with a normal but distressing colon and point out a so-called spastic colitis, or the normal kink at the splenic flexure, or a few harmless diverticula of the colon, or the perfectly normal and harmless ptosis of the colon to be found in a thin woman. This sort of thing does great harm because it causes a mildly psychotic woman to believe that all of her mental distress is arising in her colon. Then she wants something drastic done about it. If the disease is all in her nervous system she should be told that.

On saying little about a slight rise in blood pressure. Today, I feel strongly that when a woman of 60 comes in with a systolic blood pressure of 160 or 180 mm. and no symptoms, I had better not say anything. I certainly will not want to tell her that she has a hypertension. I find high pressures in so many strong, healthy women that I suspect they are almost normal.

Because of the great fear of Bright's disease, I rarely mention a trace of albumin and I do not mention a slight reduction effected by a patient's urine until I have checked the blood sugar.

Many patients become confused and frightened when they cannot understand what the physician said. If we physicians are to avoid frightening many of our patients, and leaving them feeling insecure and uncertain about their future, we must learn to talk to them in simple English speech. We must keep learning to avoid the use of our technical jargon. One day I heard one of America's most distinguished physicians say to an old farmer, "The trouble with you is that your N.P.N. is too high!" What good did that do?

Every one of us physicians must keep remembering how easy it is for a certain type of patient to misconstrue what is said to him. He may do this because of lack of intelligence or education or he may do it from a refusal to face unpleasant truths or to give up a protective illness.

Many patients easily become confused. Let us remember that if all patients were sensible and intelligent and with a retentive memory, and if all were able to grasp and understand and retain and take comfort in what was told them, matters would not be so bad; but many of our patients are dull or forgetful or apparently desirous of a bad diagnosis and a bad prognosis. Hence, they pick up eagerly and cling to any little thing that was said that could be twisted and construed into something alarming and discouraging. Persons who do this sort of thing, of course, are mildly psychotic, and many are hypochondriacal and pessimistic all their days.

On rare occasions, even when I have told a psychotic woman that all she had to explain her abdominal distress was a sore colon, or a bit of nervousness, I have had a relative come in a day or two later to ask, "Why did you frighten my sister half to death?" Or, "since you found a cancer, why didn't you go ahead to arrange for an operation?" Evidently, I had not succeeded in explaining things to the patient.

One thing is certain, and that is that we physicians who would like to help our patients, and who would like to avoid disturbing them unnecessarily should learn to speak very simply and clearly, in Anglo-Saxon English, and not in our medical shorthand.

The dangers of talking in the operating room. All surgeons and anesthetists should warn their assistants and nurses that many patients, when supposed to be under an anesthetic, can still hear and understand what is going on around them. Also, the drowsy, drugged patient lying on the operating table, waiting for the field to be prepared, can hear a lot of things which, later, may prove to be very bad for his peace of mind.

The dangers of making a vague diagnosis. Every so often a patient says, "My doctor told me I have 'weak lungs.' Just what did he mean by that? Did he mean that I am coming down with tuberculosis or am I likely to get it, or have I had it, or what?" Another patient will say, "My doctor told me I have a 'weak heart.' What did he mean by that? Is it diseased or is it going to be diseased? Or is the trouble serious?" The patient may have no mental peace until he is satisfied as to exactly what the doctor meant. Obviously, we physicians should never make such vague and meaningless and worrisome statements.

The bad results of trying to play it safe. A number of us disturb our patients by not coming out positively one way or another about a heart. We may think it is normal and we may say it is, but we may not say this definitely because we want to leave ourselves an avenue of escape. We want to play the game so that if the patient should later drop dead, we can say to the family, "Well, you remember I said that that was a definite possibility."

Because of this hedging on our part, some of us do great harm. Although, when we see a person who has a fibrositic or neurotic pain in his chest we tell him that we doubt if he has any heart disease, we advise him to ease up on work, to stop running upstairs, to give up walking, sexual intercourse, driving a car, eating meat, smoking, and taking a cocktail. All of us have known worrisome persons who, under the impact of this sort of thing, went to pieces nervously. I have had to spend years trying to get patients so treated to start living normally again.

It is true that every so often a man who has a perfectly normal electrocardiogram will drop dead. But we physicians must accept this risk, and when we find a man who has no sign of heart disease, we must say so, strongly and firmly and with conviction. If we hedge and keep open a line of retreat, we will not only fail to cure cardiac neuroses but we will make many of them.

The physician who takes refuge in silence. Many wise old physicians get so disgusted over misunderstandings with patients that they soon develop the habit of saying nothing. When asked anything, they just grunt, or they do not seem to hear anything, or they walk away. This practice, of course, has its advantages for the doctor, but it is most unsatisfactory to the patient, and it causes much hostility to doctors and the cause of medicine. It is not a good practice.

Iatrogenic disease can be due to a clerical mistake in reporting findings. I remember a young woman who came in one day almost hysterical because an eminent physician had told her she was a potential diabetic. She was so fearful because, in the pre-insulin days, several of her relatives had died in coma. The doctor had told her she had a blood sugar of 171 mg. When I found that two of her blood sugar readings were 117 mg., I got an idea, and telephoned my friend to search in his laboratory for the original figure. He soon reported that the reading was 117 mg., but his secretary had a tendency to reverse figures!

I have seen several other persons mentally hurt by this sort of thing, and the lesson all of us should learn is that all questionable reports should be held back until the test is repeated once or several times.

I remember a lovely, virginal young woman who was told she had syphilis because she got the report that should have gone to another woman of the same name. Why hadn't her physician sense enough to have the test checked and repeated before he said anything about it?

Anxieties produced by conflicting opinions. Many persons get into an awful mental state when one physician orders an immediate operation and another can find nothing the matter. To illustrate: a worrisome woman, on going for a routine cancer check-up, was told that she had a tumor of her uterus which might become cancerous and hence must be removed the very next morning. Much frightened, she went to another physician who told her she hadn't any tumor. The next one said she had a small symptomless tumor that was of no significance and needed no treatment. The next one said she had a tumor but there was no hurry about operating, and the next said there was a tumor and she should go right into the hospital. By this time the woman was in a terrible state of perplexity and anxiety.

I could not hope to put a stop to her search for some unanimity among doctors unless I could explain to her why several prominent men had differed so decidedly. I had to show her how all of them could be right according to their lights. When I examined her I found a hard uterus, about half a size too big, with a small nubbin of muscle projecting forward from the fundus. As I said, some physicians might call this a tumor, while others would not. Some physicians might fear cancer, while others would know that a myoma so rarely becomes sarcomatous that the danger of leaving it in is much less than the danger of taking it out. Some surgeons would hate to throw the woman into a menopause earlier than was necessary, and some would prefer to wait a few years for the natural menopause to take care of the situation. Some would be much influenced by the fact that she had no symptoms, while others would cling to their rule that every myomatous uterus should be removed on general principles.

I tried hard to straighten the woman out, but I doubt if I succeeded. I imagine she kept going from one doctor to another, and that eventually she gave in and accepted an operation as the only thing that would ever restore her peace of mind.

We physicians should be optimists and, when possible, should avoid making a bad prognosis. It is bad enough for a physician to make a bad prognosis when he is right. Because of it, the patient's family may hate him all their days. It is very foolish for a physician to make a bad prognosis *when no one asked him about the future.* We should all remember how many patients we have seen who refused to die quickly, as they should have done with some serious disease. The other day I saw a man alive and the picture of health 10 years after he had come to me, going blind with a malignant hypertension. At that time I had almost no hope for him, but as it has turned out, he belonged in that small group of these patients who recover perfectly after a lumbar sympathectomy. He now is devoted to me because I was the only man he saw who refused to give a hopeless prognosis.

The need for taking care in writing reports for the local physician of a patient. Many iatrogenic diseases are produced by letters which the consultant writes. Sometimes he sends the report to the home physician, putting into it some things that he certainly does not want the patient to learn about. But, commonly, the home physician, after reading the report to the patient, gives it to him. Then trouble may begin. After many unhappy experiences with such letters, I try always to write in such a way that no disaster will result if the local physician should hand the report to the patient. Actually, of course, the art of telling the physician all he needs to know, while avoiding anything alarming to the patient, is a difficult one.

Sometimes, also, although the consultant may say in his letter that he is sure that the gallstones that were found were having nothing to do with the patient's hysterical and gasless bloating, or his little stroke, this opinion is not accepted either by the physician or the patient. I have had cases in which my report was taken to a chiropractor for interpretation, and his opinion, much in conflict with mine, was the one accepted by the patient!

Obviously, the consultant must never write anything that suggests contempt or dislike of the patient. It is well never to mention the word "hysterical" since it makes a bad impression. Certainly, one must never use the word malingering, and one must never say that pain was faked. This can bring a nasty lawsuit.

Often, when one has to speak of a functional nervous disease, one can soften the blow by saying that, "After all this poor woman has been through, it is not surprising if her nerves started playing tricks with her."

The need for reading and checking all reports sent out. Many a time I have seen a young assistant sending out a letter of findings that he had not read. He did not know that even the best of secretaries can leave out that important word "not." Because of this, I check every letter of findings that goes out of my office. It would be rough on a patient to read that his disease "is . . . fatal" with the "not" left out!

On not doing much to hysterical or psychotic patients. Whenever I have to deal with a woman who has been suffering from some manifestation of hysteria, I avoid if I can little operations like a spinal puncture or a sternal puncture. Occasionally, I have seen such a minor operation produce a long-lasting headache or pain of hysterical origin. The resulting long hospitalization can be costly to the patient, and damaging to the reputation of the physician.

Illnesses produced by drugs. Often one of us physicians produces an illness by giving a patient too big a dose of some strong drug, or by leaving him too long on a drug which has unpleasant side-effects. Nowadays all of us see persons who have been laid up for weeks or months with a bad reaction to one of the antibiotics. We see women who, when about done with the menopause, are given such big doses of an estrogen that they start menstruating again. Then the doctor so fears cancer that he orders a curettage.

Often, when a patient says to his physician, "I cannot take codeine (or aspirin, or antibiotics or antihistaminics)," the doctor has so little patience with this sort of thing that he goes ahead, gives the drug, and later has good reason to rue the day. Every few months I see the bad results of refusing to accept a patient's warning of this type. It may well be that the patient who protested is a bit hysterical, but this is all the more reason for not throwing him (or her) into a "tizzy" such as might last for a month or two.

SUMMARY

Anxiety neuroses produced inadvertently by physicians are not rare. The physician should be optimistic; he should constantly be guarding his tongue, especially in the presence of a hypochondriacal type of patient, and he should never think aloud as he works his way toward a possibly alarming diagnosis. He must train his assistants and nurses to say little in the presence of anxious patients.

He should avoid mentioning findings such as a spastic colon or a trace of albumin, or a few colonic diverticula that have no significance. He must study the art of explaining things to patients in simple English so that they will understand him. Patients commonly get things all wrong.

Physicians who wish to reassure a patient must speak positively and without hedging. There is need for great care in writing reports to the home physician. One must keep constantly in mind that the letter is likely to be given to the patient. It might even some day show up in court in a damage suit where it could have a devastating effect on the jury.

9

THE UTILIZATION OF COMMUNITY
RESOURCES IN MEDICAL PRACTICE

*Marc H. Hollender, M.D.**

Basic to a consideration of the utilization of community resources is the question: What is medical practice? If it refers only to specific treatment procedures (i.e., surgery, medications, physical therapy, restriction of diet, etc.) there is no need to be concerned with community resources. If it refers, however, to a more comprehensive approach—perhaps best referred to as a program of medical *care*—the utilization of community resources is an integral part of the physician's function.

In recent years more and more physicians have come to subscribe to this broader definition of medical practice. They have done so for a variety of reasons. The pressure of numbers, in terms of the ever-increasing number of chronically ill and aged, has played a role. The development of rehabilitative procedures, especially in the fields of orthopedic surgery and physical therapy, has stimulated interest in what Rusk has referred to as the third phase of medicine. This interest was heightened by the war injured. The current focus on the psychosomatic approach to medicine has done much to shift the emphasis from an organ and its pathology to the whole person. In considering the whole person it naturally follows that community resources cannot be neglected. Finally, social workers and others, by demonstrating the value of

* The author is grateful for the help that he received in the preparation of this manuscript from Miss Josephine Taylor, Director of the Social Service Department of the Cook County Hospital; Miss Barbara J. Snoke, Assistant Director Social Service Department, Cook County Hospital and Mrs. Natalie Seltzer, Psychiatric Social Worker of the Psychiatric Clinic of the Neuropsychiatric Institute of the University of Illinois College of Medicine. The author also wishes to thank Mr. Ben L. Grossman, Director of Drexel Home (Home for Aged Jews), for many helpful suggestions.

community resources in a medical care program, have exerted an influence on physicians.

Even when there is agreement that the physician should utilize community resources, there may be divergent opinions about what these facilities have to offer. At one extreme, there are those who believe that community resources exist solely to provide financial assistance, and hence are reserved for the indigent. At the other extreme, there are those who regard all community projects as humanitarian endeavors. According to this misconception "humanitarianism" and "good" are equated, that is, to give is good regardless of how, to whom or for what. A third viewpoint, and the one which I will espouse, lies somewhere between these two extremes. According to this viewpoint, community resources are often, but not always, helpful in a variety of ways in a program of medical care.

NEEDS OF THE PATIENT

This brings us to the question: How can we determine which patients need the assistance that can be provided by community resources? For the most part such services are most beneficial to patients suffering from chronic diseases, emotional and mental disturbances and physical disabilities and the families of these patients.* It is well known that people react very differently to the stress of illness. This depends not only on the nature of the disorder and the limitations which it imposes, but on the patient's previous personality make-up, his social and work adjustments and his current life situation. An evaluation of these factors will usually help in determining which patients (and their families) will benefit from the help provided by community resources. In arriving at this determination the physician should be aware of his own reactions. There are some who, because of their tendency to overrate independence, will push patients "to pull themselves up by their own bootstraps." At the other extreme, there are those who tend to be infantilizing in their approach and hence block the independent strivings of patients.

---

* Occasionally the acutely ill patient needs such services. An example would be the woman who must make adequate provisions for her children before she can undergo an operation with some equanimity.

MEETING THE PATIENT'S NEEDS

When the patient's needs are determined, the next question is: What resources are available to provide for these needs? The answer to this varies to some extent from community to community. In larger cities there is usually a central referral service which the physician can call for the information he wants. The resources run a wide gamut. They span an age range from adoption agencies for newborns to homes for the aged. Available are rehabilitation programs, convalescent facilities, vocational guidance, social casework, foster homes and custodial institutions, to mention only a few.

After assessing the patient's needs and the resources that exist in the community, the next question is: How should a plan be worked out for or with the patient (and his family)? Certain generalizations can be made: (1) The plan should not disrupt the life of the patient any more than is necessary. (2) Due regard should be paid to the family unit. The best interests of the family should not be subjugated to those of the patient's. (3) Insofar as possible, the wishes of the patient (often dictated by emotional needs) should be respected. Compromises will have to be made and *the ideal* will have to give way to *the possible*. (4) A referral or a placement should be made in such a way that the patient understands that he is being sent to something and not pushed out. (5) The focus should be on what the patient *can* do rather than on what he cannot do.

The nature of the physician-patient relationship in this connection may be viewed in terms of the basic models described by Szasz and Hollender.[1] The first is that of *activity-passivity*. According to this model, the patient is incapable of making any judgment of his own and the physician must decide what is "good" or "bad" for him. The physician is active; the patient completely passive. This model, for example, is appropriate for the patient who has no close relative and who suffers from severe brain damage. The second model is that of *guidance—co-operation*. The patient is capable of expressing some feelings and aspirations of his own, but he turns to his physician for guidance and evinces a willingness to co-operate. The third model is that of *mutual participation*. It is favored by patients who, for various reasons, want to take care of themselves (at least in part). Here the physician serves as an expert who helps the patient to help himself.

One model is not better than another. It is rather a question of which is appropriate under given circumstances. Difficulties arise for example when a patient who strives for (and is capable of) mutual participation is treated at the level of activity-passivity, or conversely when a patient who should be treated at the level of activity-passivity is pushed toward mutual participation.

The utilization of community resources will now be considered in each of three age groups: childhood, adulthood and later life. Illustrative case histories will be presented.

CHILDHOOD

The following excerpt is from the case history of a child who became ill when he was about 20 months old.

Stanley, born January 1948, was first hospitalized for nephritis in September 1949. During the next two and one-half years he spent most of the time in the hospital, returning home for periods of never longer than a month. In view of the fact that both parents were blind and that there were two older, healthy children, it first appeared that adequate supervision of Stanley at home would not be possible. The child's physician and the hospital social worker held a conference with a worker of the Chicago Department of Welfare, who was responsible for the financial support of the children, and a worker of the Cook County Department of Welfare (Aid to the Blind). Foster home placement was ruled out because of the parents' devotion to this apparently hopelessly ill child. It was agreed that Stanley could be kept at home. Specific advice and close supervision was then given to the parents. The Chicago Department of Welfare worker provided for Stanley's needs even to the extent of seeing to it that he had games so that he would play quietly.

Today Stanley is home, doing well. He has not been hospitalized since early in 1954. With his blind father, he comes to the clinic regularly. His prognosis has been changed from "poor" to "good." The parents, at least, are convinced that the agencies' interest and co-operation kept Stanley and them going.

This brief case note illustrates a number of points. Stanley's treatment could not have been carried out without utilizing community resources unless he would have been kept in the hospital for much more prolonged periods of time than he was.

While financial assistance was essential, it was not the only thing that was provided. The parents were given advice and supervision so that they could be more comfortable in dealing with their son. The boy was given games which encouraged a type of quiet play that was consistent with the medical restrictions that had been recommended. The plan that was worked out did not disrupt the family unit. In this connection it can be stated that any plan that involves taking a child away from his parents is apt to be bitterly opposed. It does not matter whether the child is mentally retarded, physically handicapped or chronically ill. The usual bond of parent-child may be intensified by feelings of guilt. In those instances in which the parents are preoccupied with such a child to the detriment of their other children or of their own emotional health, the use of reason or injunctions will usually be of no avail in getting them to consider a placement plan. They will be able to do this only after they have had help in working out their guilt and other disturbing feelings.

Among the diseases or disabilities of childhood for which community resources provide services of value in a medical care program are cerebral palsy, rheumatic fever, diabetes mellitus, poliomyelitis, epilepsy, deafness and blindness. While with adults the focus is on rehabilitation or helping in the adjustment to limitations, with children an additional factor, the effect of the disease or disability on the process of emotional growth and development, must also be kept in mind. For example, diabetes mellitus and the measures instituted to control it stimulate reactions which may leave indelible marks or imprints on the child's developing personality. He may use his illness to manipulate his parents and thereby obtain almost constant indulgences (like a "spoiled" child). The price is the deleterious effect that this has on his physical health and his emotional maturation. In many ways the juvenile diabetic is like a person holding a two-edged sword. By manipulating his diet or his insulin, he can bring on reactions which he can use to coerce his parents. The other edge of the sword is turned inward since he injures himself (perhaps irreparably) to gain his end. When frustrated, the child can employ the same mechanism to get "revenge." The pattern of hurting himself to obtain revenge on his parents is especially dangerous for the diabetic child since he has ever available a means of immediately converting his impulse into action. The community resources that can be utilized to help the child and his parents include social casework and psychiatric services. Club groups and special camps for diabetic children may also be helpful. The emphasis in special camps is on accepting the facts of the illness while living as normal a life as possible.

The child or adolescent with rheumatic heart disease, who must limit his physical activity, is unable to use a channel of expression that has much importance during his developmental years. Josselyn[2] stated that the effect of the illness on the child's capacity to deal with problems aggressively is a blow to his psychic stability. She pointed out that while the physically healthy child gains confidence from dealing with problems aggressively, he is also afraid of punishment in the form of loss of the parent's love. This dilemma is solved, in part, by expressing aggression in physical activity. At the same time he dilutes some of the intensity of his emotional attachment and need for his parents through his relationship with his peers. The need to check aggressions, according to Josselyn, has another implication. It is a real blow to the child's self-esteem since success in active games is regarded as a badge of masculinity. The danger of aggressivity on the child's part also creates a feeling of helplessness in defending himself against the aggressions of others.

In helping the child with rheumatic fever during the convalescent period, institutions in which a team of specialists pool their effort may be of considerable benefit. This team may consist of occupational therapists, social caseworkers, social group workers, psychologists, psychiatrists, etc. Josselyn,[2] in discussing the psychiatric approach to the problems of the child with rheumatic heart disease, stated: "The goal of treatment must . . . be the resolution of the neurotic anxiety, and help in accepting the physically necessary limitations imposed by the heart condition. Because of this latter aspect, environmental manipulation is extremely important. The child needs to be stimulated to express his aggression, through physically safe outlets. . . . He also needs a situation in which either the parents or parent surrogates can offer him the security of an emotional relationship at the level to which he has regressed. Further, he needs to be encouraged gradually to grow away from the dependency upon those parent figures, in order to find for the first time, or rediscover the fact that in spite of his heart condition, the world of reality is not as dangerous as it has seemed. Thus it is imperative that the convalescent period for the cardiac be geared not only to the physical needs of the child, but equally to the total child."

After the convalescent period, the physical strain of play, the intensity of the school program and the stair climbing that is part of regular school attendance may be too much for some children. In many of our larger cities excellent special schools have been developed with programs geared to the needs of the child with rheumatic heart disease.

In the treatment of the child who is hard of hearing or deaf, a referral to a speech and hearing center may be made for a definitive evaluation. Such questions as school placement, the use of a hearing aid or the advisability of learning speech or lip reading may be considered. The recommendations are then sent to the referring physician who may use them in his future work with the child and his parents.

ADULTHOOD

The use of community resources in a medical care program for adults will now be discussed with the aid of illustrative excerpts from case histories.

With the patient who has an incurable disease, especially if it is carcinoma, there is always the danger that interest and support will be withdrawn. The physician may say, "After all, there is nothing more that I can do." Although the reasons why the cancer patient is avoided are complex, certainly one important factor is that he mobilizes feelings of helplessness in the doctor. Unfortunately, the patient who is doomed to die can least afford to be rejected. He needs to be sustained and fortified by other people. The following excerpt from a case history illustrates how community resources may be of benefit to an incurably ill or dying patient.

Mrs. L, a 50-year-old married woman of Mexican birth, was admitted to the Cook County Hospital because of an infection about her colostomy (performed six years before), but she was found to have an inoperable carcinoma of the cervix. Although the physician felt that the patient needed to be sent to a nursing home, she was so eager to return to her own apartment that a plan for her to do so was worked out by Social Service. A visiting nurse was sent out to supervise medications, dress the infected area and provide other care as needed. The patient was given morphine tablets with instructions to take them every four hours. In the hospital it had been noted that she had never asked for opiates ahead of schedule and that she got along without medication until the pain became extremely intense. The American Cancer Society furnished dressings to be used over the colostomy; the Salvation Army supplied a housekeeper five days a week and the volunteer transportation corps of the cancer society brought the patient to the clinic and the radiation center when she was able to stand the trip in a station wagon. Until that time a county physician visited her at home. After two and a half months, Mrs. L. called to say that she did not need the housekeeper any longer. She was able to be up and about, do her own cooking and go to church. She even was able to care for her colostomy herself. Church friends were willing to help her when she needed assistance. The visiting nurse thought that it would be wise to let the patient try to take this step ahead. Although rehospitalization was necessary twice between 1952 and 1955, Mrs. L. insisted on returning home each time in spite of greater pain and more marked disability. The medical social worker "stood by" to provide help as needed and many community resources were used. Mrs. L. died in the Fall of 1955.

This woman rejected a plan of placement that seemed appropriate for her physical state. Her wishes (emotional needs) were taken into consideration, and to a large extent the doctor-patient relationship was that of mutual participation. She was strongly motivated to return to her home even though this entailed considerable hardship. With help she was able to maintain herself for a three-year period. It is easy to imagine that if she had been arbitrarily placed in a nursing home that she might have become depressed or at least that her remaining years would have been less tolerable than they were. People like this patient, who are strongly motivated, who show determination and courage and who derive benefit from what is done for them evoke positive responses in those about them. They reach out and the response is one in kind. The situation is different when the person seems to more or less give up or becomes depressed or sullen. Here a much greater degree of patience and perseverance is necessary. The relationship then is usually guidance—co-operation but at times it may have to be activity-passivity. There is no display of courage by the patient with which the physician can empathize. Instead he may be appalled by the feeling of helplessness and hopelessness that is all pervasive. Often the goal in this type of situation must be extremely limited, but even then community resources may be used with benefit.

The following is a second illustrative case note.

A psychiatrist was asked to see Mrs. S., a 54-year-old woman of Lithuanian extraction, because she had talked of killing herself. It was learned that an emergency tracheotomy had been performed two days before and she was about to be discharged from the hospital with instructions to return for office visits. Mrs. S. had come to Chicago from downstate and she was completely alone in the city for the first time. In addition to the concern about her tracheotomy and what it might mean, she felt handicapped by her limited ability to speak English. She literally felt like a little girl, who was lost and frightened. This state was relieved when, on the psychiatrist's recommendation, a medical social worker provided support and assistance. The social worker made arrangements for the patient to live with a Lithuanian family, helped her get accustomed to traveling about the city and, above all, provided her with a solid "leaning post." The change in Mrs. S.'s outlook was both sudden and dramatic. In this instance the patient was called upon to assume a type of independent functioning that was beyond her emotional means. When guidance and direct help were provided she was able to co-operate in a prescribed medical program.

A third case illustration is the following.

Miss N., a 50-year-old woman, was referred for psychiatric help for a depression by her physician who had previously treated her for hypertension and urticaria. The depressed state had been mobilized by an intense, but unconscious, conflict about hostile impulses toward her employer (a mother surrogate). The patient had been working for this aged woman as a housekeeper and companion for almost 20 years. Since it was not possible in this instance to effect basic changes in the patient's personality, an effort was made to help re-establish a state of emotional equilibrium. She was hospitalized in a psychiatric unit for a brief period to remove external pressures and thereby to help her reconstitute her defenses. The assistance of a vocational guidance agency was then enlisted. After a few weeks in a sheltered workshop she was helped to find a job that was reasonably routine and secure. A sister helped in the total plan by finding the patient a room near her home and by having the patient eat some meals with her. The patient responded well and remained in a state of emotional "compensation" for three years at the end of which time she again became depressed.

In doing psychotherapy there are two approaches: (1) To effect fundamental personality changes using psychoanalysis or dynamically oriented psychotherapy, and (2) to cover over unconscious conflicts which have come closer to the surface and disrupt the patient's emotional balance. With the former approach, community resources are not used as adjunctive aids;* with the latter they may be of considerable value. This is especially true when technics such as direction and environmental manipulation are employed. The last case cited is such an instance. The goal here was to cover over the conflict rather than to resolve it. This was accomplished (for a period of three years) by removing the patient from the stressful situation and helping her to establish a new way of life.

There are, of course, many other disorders of young and middle adulthood for which community resources may be utilized in a medical care program. In the treatment of multiple sclerosis rehabilitation centers may be used to appraise and to reduce the degree of disability, the state vocational rehabilitation program offers opportunities for job retraining and social casework may be of benefit to the family of the patient. When bed care is necessary, convalescent or nursing homes may be considered.

Alcoholism is an ever-present problem in our civilization. Among the resources available for the alcoholic, the best known is Alcoholics Anonymous (A.A.). In some areas special clinics (Portal House in Chicago) undertake to treat people who have alcoholism as a prominent symptom. For more severely ill patients, private or public psychiatric hospitalization may be necessary.

In certain localities, patients with a particular disease have banded together and have formed clubs. There are Lost Chord Clubs (for laryngectomized patients), Colostomy Clubs, Ileostomy Clubs, etc. Many people derive benefit from the exchange of information and especially from the emotionally bolstering effect of the group.

THE AGED

As the aged population has increased, more and more facilities have been developed for this segment of our population. Although these facilities have not always kept stride with the needs, many community resources have been made available.

In medical practice the elderly man who has retired from work

---

* A psychoanalytic clinic, however, would be regarded as a community resource.

or the woman whose family has grown up and left home may consult the physician because of a variety of mild complaints. These may be essentially hypochondriacal in nature. In some instances with the loss of work contacts, friends and family, the focus has shifted from human relationships to the patient's own body. The goal is to refocus interest outward. There are several ways in which this can be done. For the ambulatory person, all day centers, church or temple groups or special clubs may be helpful. For those people who are confined to their apartments and alone when the weather is bad, the services of a friendly visitor may be enlisted. In other instances it may be possible to help to arrange a move to an apartment house unit for older people or to a home for the aged. For people of financial means a hotel apartment may be the solution. Here they will find a group of people in circumstances similar to their own. A social director will help them become acquainted. Evening programs are arranged for their entertainment. This resource has been utilized more and more as the number of older people has increased, and now even the finest hotels cater to them.

Many of the aged suffer from senile or arteriosclerotic dementia or so called "small strokes." The nature of their mental impairment and their social adjustment must be evaluated to determine the type of facility that should be used for them. Many of these people can continue to remain at home if the process is a mild one. Too often families feel impelled to do something and as a result they make changes that make matters worse rather than better. It is not an easy task to get relatives to leave well enough alone. A mildly confused person, when confronted by a new setting which calls upon him for a task of mastery beyond his mental means, may become much more confused and disturbed. In some instances the provision of a housekeeper or companion is a good solution. There are other aged people with organic brain damage who can maintain themselves in hotel apartments, homes for the aged or apartment house units for the aged. When the process is moderately advanced, nursing home placement may be a solution. In the severe cases, hospitalization in a private or state facility is necessary. When the physician consults with the family in such a situation the model of the relationship may be either guidance—co-operation or mutual participation. When it seems apparent that the family has much guilt, the former model is usually appropriate. The physician points out that the patient *must* be sent to a hospital because his illness is of such a nature that it is no longer safe for him to remain at home. It can be added that the family has no real choice since the course that must be followed is clearly dictated by the nature of the process. An honest statement of this sort, to some extent, takes the burden of guilt off the family.

Another problem with older persons arises when there is a physical disability and the question of rehabilitation is under consideration. Even though a wave of overoptimism has characterized the recent approach to the aged, there are still those situations in which the recuperative powers of some people are underestimated. The following two case notes will serve as illustrations.

A 66-year-old man had an amputation of his right leg for diabetic gangrene. When the physician told him that he would be able to go home soon, the patient asked: "How are you going to send me home?" When he was informed that the plan was to have him go in a wheel chair, he balked and said: "I'm not going that way. I am going to walk out of this hospital." Some weeks later, with a good-fitting prosthesis which he had been instructed to use, he did walk out of the hospital— and much to the pleasure of the physician who initially had underestimated his potential for rehabilitation.

Mrs. F., an 81-year-old woman, was hospitalized following a cerebrovascular accident that affected her right leg and arm. Her niece urged the physician to institute a program of rehabilitation even though he considered it a waste of effort. Physical therapy was started. At this time the patient was confused, often failed to recognize her relatives, ate poorly and spoke in a mumbled and sometimes incoherent way. She was sent from the hospital to a home for the aged where the rehabilitation program was continued. When her sensorium cleared in about four to six weeks, she expressed a desire to continue with the program. After about six months she was even able to walk a little without a walker, and she derived pleasure in showing how well she could do.

FAILURE TO UTILIZE COMMUNITY FACILITIES

There are a number of reasons why patients may fail to utilize community resources even when the physician has made an effort to get them to do so. Some of these will now be considered.

The way in which the referral is made by the physician will partly determine the patient's attitude. If the patient feels that he is being pushed out rather than sent to something, he will be resentful. If he is not presented with a clear picture of what to expect, he is especially apt to conjure up or to cling to unrealistic fantasies of what he will receive. When the fantasies fail to materialize, he becomes disappointed and disinterested. This can be illustrated by considering the referral of a child to a speech and hearing center. When the parents do not have a clear picture of what to expect they may come with unrealistic expectations. When no miracle happens, they may become disappointed and drop out after a visit or two.

A failure to utilize community resources may be the result of a patient's attempt to deny the existence of illness. A 53-year-old man, who denied that he had a cardiac disorder, returned to a job involving heavy work in spite of his physician's recommendation that he obtain other employment. He soon became decompensated and returned to the hospital. Often the approach to such a patient is to attempt to frighten him into taking a lighter job. The assumption is that he will then avail himself of the state vocational rehabilitation service or some other program for retraining. It should be understood, however, that the denial mechanism is an unconscious response designed to fend off fear and anxiety. Therefore, the approach should be to relieve enough fear and anxiety so that the patient can face the situation and make a more realistic adjustment to it.

There are other patients who refuse assistance because of intense emotional needs to be self-sufficient. They maintain patterns of overcompensatory "independence" at all cost. When this is so, psychotherapy may help them to accept help in a rehabilitation program. This subject was discussed in a recent article by Alger and Rusk.[3]

SUMMARY

When medical practice assumes a comprehensive approach, helping the patient to utilize community resources is an integral part of the physician's function. More and more physicians have come to subscribe to this broader definition. There are still divergent opinions, however, as to what community resources have to offer. One viewpoint is that they are often, but not always, helpful in a variety of ways. In planning, it is important to evaluate the patient's needs and to investigate the existing facilities in a given area. In this connection certain generalizations can be made: (1) The plan should not disrupt the life of the patient any more than is necessary. (2) While due regard should be paid to the family unit, the best interests of the family should not be subjugated to those of the patient's. (3) Insofar as possible, the emotional needs of the patient should be considered. (4) A referral or placement should be made in such a way that the patient realizes that he is being *sent to* and *not away* from something. (5) The focus should be on what the patient can do rather than on what he cannot do.

The utilization of community resources has been considered in each of three age groups: childhood, adulthood and later life. Illustrative case histories have been presented. Finally, the reasons why patients fail to utilize community resources have been discussed. If the patient believes that he is being sent away from, rather than to, something that will help him, he will be resentful. This may interfere with his co-operation in a program that would be of benefit to him. If the patient is not presented with a clear picture of what to expect, he is especially apt to conjure up or to cling to unrealistic fantasies of what he will derive. When these fantasies fail to materialize, he may quickly lose interest and drop out. There are, also, those people who because of a need to deny the existence of an illness or because of a need to be completely self-sufficient will not accept help. Psychotherapy will sometimes be of benefit to these people, and, moreover, it may make it possible for them to utilize community resources which they had previously rejected.

BIBLIOGRAPHY

1. Szasz, T. S., and Hollender, M. H.: A contribution to the philosophy of medicine. The basic models of the physician-patient relationship, A.M.A. Arch. Int. Med. 97:585-592, 1956.
2. Josselyn, Irene M.: Emotional implications of rheumatic heart disease in children, Am. J. Orthopsychiat. 19:87, 1949.
3. Alger, I., and Rusk, H. A.: The rejection of help by some disabled people, Arch. Phys. Med. 36:277, 1955.

INDEX

147